Mar. 2016

THE PARENT'S GUIDE TO
OCCUPATIONAL
THERAPY for AUTISM
and Other Special Needs

of related interest

Once Upon a Touch…
Story Massage for Children
Mary Atkinson and Sandra Hooper
ISBN 978 1 84819 287 4
eISBN 978 0 85701 234 0

The Autism Fitness Handbook
An Exercise Program to Boost Body Image, Motor Skills, Posture and
Confidence in Children and Teens with Autism Spectrum Disorder
David S. Geslak
ISBN 978 1 84905 998 5
eISBN 978 0 85700 963 0

The Asperkid's Game Plan
Extraordinary Minds, Purposeful Play…Ordinary Stuff
Jennifer Cook O'Toole
ISBN 978 1 84905 959 6
eISBN 978 0 85700 779 7

**Speak, Move, Play and Learn with
Children on the Autism Spectrum**
Activities to Boost Communication Skills, Sensory Integration
and Coordination Using Simple Ideas from Speech and
Language Pathology and Occupational Therapy
*Lois Jean Brady, America X Gonzalez,
Maciej Zawadzki and Corinda Presley*
ISBN 978 1 84905 872 8
eISBN 978 0 85700 531 1

Challenge Me!™
Mobility Activity Cards
Amanda Elliott
ISBN 978 1 84310 497 1

Motivate to Communicate!
300 Games and Activities for Your Child with Autism
Simone Griffin and Dianne Sandler
ISBN 978 1 84905 041 8
eISBN 978 0 85700 215 0

A Brief Guide to Autism Treatments
Elisabeth Hollister Sandberg and Becky L. Spritz
ISBN 978 1 84905 904 6
eISBN 978 0 85700 650 9

THE PARENT'S GUIDE TO
OCCUPATIONAL
THERAPY for AUTISM
and Other Special Needs

Practical Strategies for Motor Skills,
Sensory Integration, Toilet Training,
and More

CARA KOSCINSKI

Jessica Kingsley *Publishers*
London and Philadelphia

First edition published in 2013
This edition published in 2016
by Jessica Kingsley Publishers
73 Collier Street
London N1 9BE, UK
and
400 Market Street, Suite 400
Philadelphia, PA 19106, USA

www.jkp.com

Library of Congress Cataloging in Publication Data
Names: Koscinski, Cara author.
Title: The parent's guide to occupational therapy for autism and other
  special needs : practical strategies for motor skills, sensory
  integration, toilet training, and more / Cara Koscinski.
Other titles: Pocket occupational therapist for families of children with
  special needs
Description: Second edition. | London ; Philadelphia : Jessica Kingsley
  Publishers, 2016. | Revision of: Pocket occupational therapist for
  families of children with special needs. 2013. | Includes index.
Identifiers: LCCN 2015035761 | ISBN 9781785927058 (alk. paper)
Subjects: LCSH: Occupational therapy for children. | Children with
  disabilities.
Classification: LCC RJ53.O25 K67 2016 | DDC 615.8/515083--dc23 LC record
available at
http://lccn.loc.gov/2015035761

British Library Cataloguing in Publication Data
A CIP catalogue record for this book is available from the British Library

ISBN 978 1 78592 705 8
eISBN 978 1 78450 258 4

Printed and bound in the United States

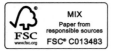

"Shoot for the moon. For even if you miss,
you'll land among the stars"

—unknown

Never underestimate the ability of
a child with special needs.

Contents

Introduction

Early in my career as an occupational therapist, I had no idea that the training I was receiving would prepare me for my personal journey. As I watched my first son grow, I noticed he showed signs of severe delays in the areas of social and emotional development. He began to miss milestones, have severe tantrums, and became more and more distant. I felt helpless and afraid. I asked questions and received no answers. When my second son came along, I knew both of my sweet children were different than other children their age. Soon, they were both diagnosed with autism spectrum disorders, sensory processing disorder, mitochondrial disease, and feeding difficulties, among others. The following years brought a grueling therapy schedule and emotional rollercoaster. I know what it's like to live with children who struggle to function with everyday tasks. I have felt the absolute joy when a tiny milestone is reached and I've felt the heartbreaking agony of defeat and rejection. It's NOT easy, but having someone to take you by the hand is important.

As I write my books, it's important to me that everyone benefits. There is no technical jargon or complicated wording and each question is answered in easy-to-understand terms. The book provides a comprehensive list of difficulties commonly seen in children who have special needs. Even parents of typically developing children can find help with behavior, sensory issues, and development. During a recent interview, someone suggested my books should be kept in the bathroom as mandatory reading. I'm OK with that. (Thanks, Shannon!)

I wrote this book as a *pocket guide* for parents. I wanted to be the OT that was there, in your pocket, when you needed answers. So, I called myself *The Pocket Occupational Therapist.* Each section answers one of the most frequently asked questions I've heard as a pediatric therapist. The topics are vast and it's my hope that you can use the book as a handy reference guide. Each question is followed by "Out of the POCKET Tips" that you can complete with your own child to help him to achieve his goals. There are many activities from which to choose and they are easy to implement at home.

The book should be used often. Topics range from sensory processing to handwriting to toileting. Also, I've covered behavior and transitions. As a mom and OT, I attend as many trainings and courses as possible. As a result, my experience is well-rounded and vast. If a technique did not work for me or my clients, I did not include it in my book. The activities are tried and true and I personally have applied them to my own children.

Thank you for joining me on the journey of raising a child with special needs. I promise, you will receive immense joy as you watch your child reach his goals. I hope you enjoy my book as much as I've enjoyed writing it.

One day at a time...

With love,

Cara

Chapter 1

What Is Occupational Therapy? My Child Doesn't Work!

What is occupational therapy and what training does an OT have?

Occupational therapy is a unique profession that designs a plan of treatment specifically for each person as an individual with unique physical, emotional, social, psychological, and cultural needs. The slogan for occupational therapy has become "skills for the job of living." Disabilities, illnesses, and special needs affect each person differently and a treatment plan for occupational therapy includes that person's specific goals.

The occupational therapist (OT) has specific training in a wide variety of areas. Some of these include: human development, psychology, sociology, anatomy, neurology, physiology, and kinesiology (the study of movement). There are programs that include the dissection of parts of cadavers (human bodies) as a means to fully understand the physical structure of humans. During the course of study, the OT student must fulfill specific requirements of study in an actual clinical setting. This is called "fieldwork" and you may encounter a student therapist during your child's treatment. The requirements for training are set forth by a governing body and each college offering a degree in OT is accredited.

There are times when an OT Assistant may work with your child. The training of OT Assistants is unique as they are specifically trained in implementing the treatment plan designed by the OT. The OT Assistant is creative in planning activities to help a child meet her therapy goals. In the USA, the training for an Assistant lasts for two years and results in an Associate's Degree. OT Assistants are not permitted to write a treatment plan, assess, or formulate goals without the supervision of the OT. They must also complete clinical training in addition to the classroom work. The OT Assistant and OT are a wonderful complement to each other's skills.

I am often asked why it looks as if I'm only playing with a child during my session. The occupation of a child is to play. Children learn through the completion of activities that they perform on a daily basis. By learning that their actions cause a reaction, either by a toy or human, they experience a feeling of success. When an activity is successful, it is likely to be repeated. In the same way, when a child has failed during an activity, he may not want to do the activity again. He may have a feeling of failure with repeated unsuccessful attempts. Occupational therapists are specifically trained to use age-appropriate activities to work on the development of skills that are used in daily life. This means that an OT working with children is able to choose play activities and games that are at the child's specific developmental level so that success can be accomplished. When a child is successful at a new skill, it is the goal of the OT to ensure that the child is able to build on that skill. When a child has not been able to succeed at a skill, he must be given the chance to complete it. With success comes pleasure and it is an OT's job to plan activities in which your child is able to succeed and have fun at the same time.

What do all of those initials mean after my OT's name?

There are OTs who have Bachelor's degrees practicing in the USA today, but as of 2007 all OTs who graduated had either a Master's or professional Doctoral degree. Initials you may see after your therapist's name, particularly in the USA, may include:

- *OTR* = Occupational Therapist, Registered by the NBCOT (National Board of Certification of Occupational Therapists)

- *OTR/L* = Occupational Therapist Registered by the NBCOT and Licensed in the state where they work

- *MA* = Master of Arts

- *MS* = Master of Science

- *MOT* = Master of Occupational Therapy

- *OTD* = Occupational Therapy Doctorate

- *FAOTA* = Fellow of the American Occupational Therapy Association

- *COTA* = Certified Occupational Therapy Assistant.

What is ADL?

ADL stands for Activities of Daily Living. Activities of daily living are simply the things that someone does in their everyday life. Adults get dressed, work, cook, clean, are caregivers, drive, and complete recreational activities. Children do most of the same things that adults do such as dressing and bathing, but the work of a child is to play. When a child plays, he learns valuable skills that he will use as an adult. So, playing activities are practice for grown-up tasks such as setting up a store, playing house, working with pretend tools, and so on.

An OT looks at a child's activities from the time she wakes up until she goes to bed. Every activity may be impacted differently by the child's area of weakness. If a child has low tone in her trunk, sitting in a chair to eat breakfast, participating in gym class, and riding in the car may all be affected. The occupational therapist is trained to use play activities specifically designed to improve areas of a child's weaknesses. This is why your child's therapy session looks like play. One of the greatest comments I receive in my sessions is "My child looks as if she is having a good time!" A child is much more likely to learn while she is enjoying the process.

What makes an OT different from other therapists?

The OT is uniquely trained in activity analysis. This means looking at the specific parts of an activity in order to determine its effects and demands on the person who is completing it. Analysis of an activity is the main tool of occupational therapy, since occupational therapy practitioners are called upon to help their patients with daily activities following a disease or if they have a disability. Here is an example of activity analysis:

Activity: Write the Letter "A"

Steps:

1. Grasp the writing utensil (pencil) with your hand.

2. Hold the pencil with your muscles tightly enough to keep it in your hand.

3. Use the right amount of pressure to make a mark on the paper.

4. Form the letter correctly—this part requires many different strokes of the pencil as each letter must be made by thinking about its shape and then using the muscles to make the appropriate motion.

As you can see, there are many steps to writing just ONE letter. What if your child had difficulty with grasping the pencil or forming the correct shape to make part of the A...? We could go on further, but the point is that OTs don't make any assumptions about activities; they look at the child's weak area and then analyze the steps that the child must take to achieve success. After recognizing the problem, a specific goal must be made to help fix it.

Occupational therapists specifically look at how each special need affects the child's life and helps to problem-solve with the caregivers. A unique relationship with the treatment team results. There are also times when the therapist who usually works in an outpatient clinic setting or school may travel to the child's home to fully determine how the child's function is impacted in various environments.

How do I choose the right OT for my child?

The first thing to determine is that your occupational therapist has graduated from an AOTA-accredited program or equivalent if you are outside the USA.[1] The AOTA stands for the American Occupational Therapy Association. Their website (www.aota.org) is a wonderful resource that has a specialist directory on the site. Membership in the AOTA is not mandatory for occupational therapists in the USA, but attending and graduating from an AOTA-accredited school is mandatory for taking the board certification exam required to become an OT.

The National Board of Certification in Occupational Therapy (NBCOT) requires that every OT passes an examination that they design and moderate upon graduating from college. The exam is given at specific locations and passing the exam gives the OT a certification called OTR or Occupational Therapist, Registered. Most US states require that a therapist carries a license in the state in which the OT practices. In order to receive that license, the OT must have passed the OTR examination. Regular continuing education must be completed by the OT and certificates are submitted to the national board and/or state licensure board.

It is also important to choose a therapist who will answer any questions you have about their training,

---

1   A list of international associations that award occupational therapy accreditation can be found at the end of this book.

methods of treatment, and special interests. It is critical that your OT be a good personality match with your child. You may be working with the OT for a long period of time and want to have good communication about your goals for your child. The OT must complete a thorough assessment of your child's abilities and areas of weakness. Specific goals should be made for your child and reviewed with you. I encourage you to obtain a copy of your child's assessment and treatment goals. Regular re-evaluations should be completed to make sure that progress in the goal areas is being made. If your OT isn't willing to discuss progress and ways he is trying to achieve your child's goals in each session, you may with to consider a change of therapist.

Energy in the session and a positive attitude is critical for success in therapy. I once hired an OT with excellent training, expensive and extensive continuing education, and an impressive résumé. She interviewed well but during her trial employment she demonstrated a lack of excitement during her sessions. Smiling, clapping, and general encouraging words along with a willingness to be flexible and adapt to your child's needs are all critical to successful goal achievement. As with any profession, someone may look wonderful on paper, but may behave totally differently when presented with challenges. For this reason, I encourage you to sit in or request to be a silent observer in the first few sessions to ensure a good fit. A word of caution, though: do not interrupt the therapist during the session, but instead wait until afterwards to discuss concerns and issues regarding goals. It is extremely important to respect everyone's time.

A good fit would be someone who you feel truly listens to your concerns and to your child's communication style. Often, the therapist is working on non-preferred (difficult) skills. There may be periods when your child becomes frustrated when learning and the therapist should know how to motivate him to have fun while learning at the same time. Since the OT will only be working with your child one or two times per week, it is important to have good communication about activities that you may do at home to carry over the treatment in the clinic or school setting. I loved giving my caregivers "homework" for the week and enjoyed hearing how proud the child was to show his hard work!

What does "SIPT certified" or "SIPT certification" mean?

If you suspect that your child has difficulty with sensory processing, it is important to ask your OT if he has experience and special training in this area. You may hear that a therapist is "SIPT certified." The pronunciation is "sipped." This means that he has attended a special training in administering the Sensory

Integration Praxis Test. This unique series of tests was created by A. Jean Ayres PhD, OTR, FAOTA, an OT who developed the theory of the sensory integration framework. It was Dr. Ayres who developed and published the SIPT (Sensory Integration and Praxis Test) in 1989—sold through Western Psychological Services. There is an older version of the SIPT called SCSIT or Southern California Sensory Integration Tests which was published in 1972.

It is not mandatory that your OT be SIPT certified. In fact, sensory processing research and terminology continues to evolve over time. Many therapists seek training, mentorship, and continuing education courses in sensory processing disorders. Parents can also attend conferences designed to help their child with SPD. A great resource is the SPD Foundation at www. SPDFoundation.net.

Note: It is advisable to consult your child's doctor before trying any of the activities in this book.

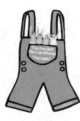

Out of the POCKET Activity

Things to determine about your new OT:

- What is her specialty and what extra training does she have in that area?

- What does her typical treatment session involve? Is it fun for your child while working on specific goals?

- Does she give homework for you each week to carry over your child's goals?

- Does she complete a thorough evaluation targeting sensory AND daily living skills?

- Does she listen to you and answer your questions?

- Is the OT working on goals that are important to your family and to your child?

I have two instances when I have had to request a different OT for my son. First, I felt the OT was not a good match for him. He needed an energetic therapist with a structured setting. The OT was fun, but did not utilize structure. This did not work for my son's specific learning style. The second therapist was not trained in any feeding techniques and had little experience in feeding therapy. I was willing to switch days and times and requested an OT more experienced in feeding. The scheduling department had given me the first available therapist instead of considering my child's specific needs. Occupational therapists want your child to progress as much as you do—no one wants to waste time. You are your child's best advocate and know her specific needs. Do not be afraid to discuss your goals and progress with your child's OT.

What is in an occupational therapy report and should I ask to see my child's report?

When you decide to take your child to an occupational therapist, it is important to know what areas the therapist will be assessing or testing. The OT is skilled at giving special tests that look at key areas of development. There are assessments designed for looking at handwriting; developmental skills such as writing, cutting, holding blocks, and tossing a ball; sensory processing activities and function; body position such as a baby's ability to sit, crawl, or roll; and even tests for specific muscle strength. A therapist who specializes in working with children with autism should be competent in assessing sensory processing and how it affects a child's function in everyday life.

The OT will discuss your concerns about your child with you. Then, tests will be selected to get an objective (or concrete and not skewed) developmental or skill level. You should be asked specific developmental questions about when your child sat up, rolled, fed himself, used the toilet, began talking, and met milestones that are generally expected to occur. (A checklist of these milestones is given at the end of this book.) The caregiver's input, responses, and cooperation in the assessment and therapy process may directly affect the outcome of therapy.

After the evaluation is completed, which usually takes about an hour for most children, your OT will write a report of her findings. You should get a copy of the report and discuss it with the therapist. Often, therapists' schedules are tight so you might want to request a specific time to talk together. The report usually begins with the reason you brought your child in, the prescribing physician's name, and then outlines your child's developmental history. There will be an overview of his general body strength in his core and arms. Look for any terms you do not understand and request an explanation of them. For example, MMT stands for Manual Muscle Testing, which is a general standard in assessing the strength of specific muscles or groups of muscles.

There will be a section about how independently your child dresses, bathes, buttons, zips, ties shoes, uses the toilet, positions her body for activities of daily living, and her current functional level. Cognition is assessed in the report. Cognition involves our ability to pay attention, remember, follow directions, and orient ourselves to the time and place. The area of cognition is important in looking at your child's ability to participate in daily tasks. OTs are trained at assessing and working on improving cognition in relation to activities of daily living.

The assessment section is the area of the report where the therapist sums up her findings and places them into a nice little package of a few sentences in order to discuss the areas of weakness and strengths, and to prepare for the goal-setting process. Finally, the goal list is the specific target areas with measurable outcomes. Goals will be monitored frequently by the OT and will be updated when needed. It is important that you understand your child's specific goals as you will be investing a lot of your time in traveling, attending, and working on carryover of therapy.

Chapter 2

What Are Core Muscles and Reflexes and Why Are They Important to My Child's Function?

What is a core muscle?

Core muscles are those muscles in the abdomen and mid- and lower-back. They support the spine and run the length of the torso (the trunk or part of the body without arms and legs). Core muscles are so important in our daily lives because when they contract they support the spine, pelvis, and shoulder to give us a solid base of support. It is difficult to visualize these muscles because some of them are deep in our bodies. Sometimes I encourage parents to imagine that they are having a bowel movement...the contraction of the core muscles can be felt at that time. The core muscles have the additional job of protecting our organs and helping us with balance, posture, and stability. Most often, we look at a fitness class doing push-ups or sit-ups that will strengthen their core or tone their bodies. Yoga instructors emphasize core muscle strengthening.

What should my therapist look for to assess core muscles?

Strong core muscles are crucial to providing us with a good base of support. I cannot tell you how many times children have come to my clinic after working with other therapists who have not assessed their child's core musculature weaknesses. When your child is lacking in core muscle stability and strength, many problems with completing everyday tasks may result. Some areas of weakness may include: poor handwriting, difficulty sitting at a desk for long periods of time, poor posture or slumping, inability to ride a bicycle, and difficulty with skipping and hopping.

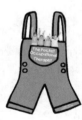

Out of the POCKET Activity

Every child who I work with is tested in the following ways to determine core strength:

- Can he do push-ups and sit-ups?

- How long can he stand on one foot?

- Can he skip, do jumping jacks, and hop?

- Can he walk on a taped line with a tight heel-to-toe pattern?

- How is his posture during handwriting activities or activities requiring him to be seated in a chair at a table?

- Can he lie on his stomach and then slowly lift his arms and legs up into a "superman" position?

- Can he ride a bicycle with two wheels when age-appropriate?

What does handwriting have to do with core muscle weakness?

Without a good base of support, a child may have difficulty with prolonged use of the arms and legs. Let's think about a child in school all day. She must sit at her desk for long periods of time. If she has a weak core, she may begin her day sitting upright in her chair, but as time passes she fatigues quickly and begins to slump onto her desk. When she must complete paper and pencil tasks, she is already tired and lacks the energy to use her arms. I encourage you to attempt to write a paragraph while slumped over at your desk. It is truly difficult.

Humans need a good strong base of support in our trunk to complete tasks with our arms and hands. The core muscles support the shoulder muscles, which then support the arm muscles, which support the hand musculature…it's like a pyramid that needs a strong base. If the base is weak, then the rest crumbles immediately or can only support the top for a brief period. You can ask your child's teacher about her posture at her desk or notice her posture during homework time in the evening. Also, do your own "assessment" and ask her to write a paragraph in her best handwriting and take note of her body position while writing at the beginning and end of the assignment.

What is "W" sitting?

Your child may sit with his legs in a "W" formation. His legs literally look like a W when you look down at him sitting on the floor. Children sit in this way because they seek a bigger base of support for their bodies due to low tone and weak core musculature and can create this support with their legs. It's a lot harder to sit "criss-cross applesauce" than to "W" sit if you have weak muscles in your trunk. I encourage you to "W" sit and note how much more difficult it is for you to take in a deep breath in this slouched position. When you "W" sit, note how your hips/pelvic girdle tilt backwards, causing your shoulders to come forward. This position is not good for working on speech sounds requiring sustained breath and encourages bad posture.

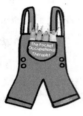

Out of the POCKET Activity

When you notice your child "W" sitting, encourage him to sit "criss-cross applesauce." Give him a cue when you notice him "W" sitting. It may be helpful to demonstrate this position and sit with him to play a game. Begin with a short activity and progress to longer ones so that your child can be successful when sitting. Core muscles take time to become strong and working at your child's pace is important for success.

Why is "tummy time" so important for my child?

The "Back to Sleep" campaign may have lessened the incidence of SIDS (Sudden Infant Death Syndrome), but as parents we need to remember to encourage "tummy time" to work on our children's core musculature. A child without special needs may have the ability to roll over more quickly than a child with low tone or with poor coordination. Our children with weak muscles need to work harder to develop their core and work against gravity while on their bellies. "Tummy time" should always be supervised with your baby, but is a crucial activity for developing those core muscles. I encourage caregivers to place the baby on his tummy and then use a brightly colored toy or one with music to attract his attention. Begin with short periods of time and work up at his own pace. He will slowly learn to raise his head against gravity and further develop his ability to use his arms and legs while on his stomach. You will be proud of yourself for helping your child's development!

Why is crawling so important?

We often don't consider the importance of crawling to our development. In fact, crawling refines both gross and fine motor skills. Crawling helps to develop shoulder stability as the infant uses her arms to bear weight. It helps a child to learn balance of the arm, legs, and trunk. The movements of crawling send information to the brain from tactile (touch), visual (sight), and proprioception (deep muscle) receptors. A child must use her eyes together to focus on the area she's exploring, and must use her neck muscles to support her head. Her vestibular system (which affects position in space) is receiving information and practicing for the movements of walking and running. The reciprocal movements of the arms and legs involve coordination of the large muscle groups for bilateral integration. Bilateral integration is when the body uses both sides together to accomplish a task. Author Carla Hannaford's book *Smart Moves* frequently refers to movement as it plays a critical role in development of nerve cell networks required for learning throughout the lifespan.

During crawling, the pressure of the hands on the floor helps to develop the arches of the hand and stretch out ligaments, which are crucial to fine motor tasks such as handwriting. To demonstrate, think of the tightness of a newborn baby's hand and imagine how it needs to stretch and eventually become refined and flexible enough to pick up the smallest item from the table. Try touching your thumb to the tip of your pinky finger (the finger furthest from the thumb). One of the arches in your hands allows it to make the "cupping" that results from that movement. In children who cannot crawl due to physical limitations, it is imperative that the OT give him chances to develop the muscles by the use of adapted activities. These activities should include opportunities to bear weight through the arms and hands.

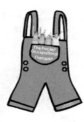

Out of the POCKET Activity

In my practice, I always implement "tummy time" with my clients. The activity you choose should be arranged so that your child has no idea that she is doing exercise/work. Start by asking your child to lie on her stomach while playing, but ensure that she doesn't fatigue too quickly and become frustrated. If your child cannot complete any activity while on her stomach, then use a bean bag or pillows to make a wedge to support her trunk. As your sessions progress, make the games longer, such as a game of Go-Fish, and add more arm movements while in this position. Hand-clapping games are fun too. What is especially motivating for children is to see their entire family lying on their tummies to play a game together!

You will sometimes see your OT work on "tummy time" with the use of a therapy swing. Again, the child lies on his stomach on the swing and works against gravity to pick up bean bags and then toss them around the room to the OT. This activity is especially popular with my male clients who love throwing things at different targets. I have even put up dart boards and have scattered the darts around the room. The child propels himself in the swing to pick up the darts one at a time.

Crawling in therapy is a wonderful activity to provide input and work on strengthening of gross and fine motor skills. Make an obstacle course for your child. Be sure to include tunnels or crawling under tables for more input. Walking on hands and feet like a crab is where the child reaches backwards with hands on the floor behind her back and tries to keep her bottom off the floor. She can also try to kick a ball from this position. Wheelbarrow walking is when you hold your child's feet and have her crawl on the floor using her hands.

Any of these activities will be difficult for children who have difficulty getting into the crawling position. Make sure to start slowly and progress gradually. An OT will tell you that a child must work up from brief periods of activity to more prolonged ones. Your child will be more likely to play the games in positions that are difficult for him if you get involved and make the games fun. Try to work together and be sure to ask your therapist for advice on which activities to begin with.

What does positioning mean?

In order to complete fine motor or skilled tasks involving the hands, we need a base of support. Our core muscles provide the base of support we need to be successful using our hands. Positioning with the feet flat on the floor is important while completing seated tasks. We should sit in our chairs with our thighs parallel to the floor, our back should be comfortably resting vertically on the chair, and our forearms should be resting on the table parallel to the floor. We call this a 90–90–90 position. The result is a 90-degree angle at our ankles, knees, and hips. If a child is slouching in his chair, he will quickly fatigue when using his hands.

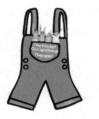

Out of the POCKET Activity

To help with positioning of the wrist and hands at the table during handwriting, an inclined surface works well. Use a three-ring binder that's four inches wide. Place the paper on a clipboard on top of the binder. The use of the binder provides an inclined surface which helps with positioning of the hand and wrist for handwriting.

Your child should be permitted to rest her forearms on the table for greater stability when using her fingers.

How does a baby develop the ability to move while in the womb?

When a baby is in the womb, he is floating in a gravity-free environment. His body is surrounded by amniotic fluid. The fluid allows the baby to practice breathing and swallowing, helps the womb to stay at a consistent temperature, and provides protection from the bumps that occur from the outside world. One of the biggest benefits of being surrounded by fluid is that baby can practice moving necessary to develop stronger bones and muscles. While in the womb babies suck their thumbs, play with their own feet, and even kick against the placenta. Practicing movements helps build coordination that baby will need once he enters the outside world. Additionally, an unborn baby responds to his mother's voice! Many tests have shown that a newborn baby's heart rate slows down when hearing mom's voice. What's more exciting is that a baby *in utero* responds when his face, lips, and cheeks are touched. He begins to move toward the stimulus with his mouth open. This means that baby is developing the rooting reflex. When a baby is born, he needs the rooting reflex to turn toward mom's breast. Anytime a baby's cheek is brushed or stroked, he reflexively turns toward that cheek with his mouth open, ready to feed.

What are reflexes?

A new baby has many "built-in" mechanisms to help him to move against gravity. Most of us know that when your doctor taps his hammer on the front of your knee, he's looking for the knee-jerk reflex. We are hard-wired with reflexes which protect us from danger. For example, when you touch a hot stove, your body automatically withdraws your hand. This reflex happens so quickly that we don't even have time to think about it. Similarly, a baby is born with reflexes which help her learn to eat, grasp, protect herself from loud noises, and move. As baby repeats the reflexive movements over and over, she gets stronger and her movements become purposeful; in essence the reflex fades away. So, many reflexes help baby to learn purposeful movements and disappear as baby develops more movements on her own. One of the best things is that OTs can help baby use reflexes to work on developing purposeful coordinated movements through play-based activities. When babies learn to walk, there is no "switch" that comes on randomly. Baby slowly learns to stand, balance, and contract muscles to shift weight between her legs. Many moms get excited that their babies can "walk." Babies reflexively step when their bare feet touch the floor. It is an amazing sight to see a two-month old baby, who is otherwise helpless, march her legs. However, therapists know that this is simply a reflex over which baby has no control and the reflex disappears around three months of age. It's similar to our knee-jerk reaction, but is designed to help baby develop coordination in preparation for purposeful walking movement. So, some reflexes disappear and some, such as blinking our eyes, stay with us for life.

Why do parents need to know about reflexes?

Recently, there has been a lot of talk about reflexes and the lack of movement opportunities for baby. Many "containers" designed to hold baby up or transport her during a parent's busy life have decreased baby's opportunity to freely move and experience the environment. Car seats, props, cushions, baby walkers, bouncy chairs, and the like restrict movement OR force baby to rely on muscles which are not ready to mature. A baby is designed to progress and develop through a specific set of milestones. Inhibition of sensory or movement experiences in one stage may hinder developmental progression in the future. For example, soft infant seats (I'll refrain from naming a brand) are designed to prop a young baby up to "see" her environment. However, babies younger than six months are generally not ready to sit up for a prolonged period. The baby is restricted in her movement while in the chair and can fatigue easily. Her body does not yet have the head and postural control required to sit. In fact, head control is best developed through periods of "tummy time." When baby is ready to sit, she will do so and it is critical to follow your baby's developmental signs. There is simply no substitute for sensory and movement play which is supervised by an adult. Allowing baby to move helps to integrate reflexes and mature her body for later tasks. If a baby does not move through the natural progression of movement and reflex integration, she may experience difficulty later in life.

Parents benefit from the knowledge about reflexes and the progression of motor and sensory development of baby. Understanding that primitive reflexes have a limited life-span and should have integrated into controlled and purposeful movements is important. When a child has a retained reflex, or one that has remained longer than it should, the parents can pick up on some cues that therapy may be needed. For example, if a five-year-old typically developing child reflexively grasps his mother's hand as an infant does (palmar grasp reflex), there may be a problem since the reflex should have disappeared by four months of age. Trauma or other problems may manifest themselves in the reappearance of reflexes. Another example is the Moro (startle) reflex. When a baby hears loud noises, feels unexpected movement, or he has the sensation of falling, he cries while extending his arms, legs, and fingers. His back then arches and he retracts his arms and legs. Moro is the baby's first independent attempt at protecting himself. It should be fully integrated and disappear by six months of age. There are many websites which discuss infant reflexes and the integration process. Information about reflexes can provide critical clues to parents about their child. When any reflex is retained later that it should be, please discuss this with the pediatrician or therapist.

Chapter 3

Feeding and Oral-Motor (Muscles of the Mouth)

Feeding problems are some of the most difficult and long-lasting issues that occupational therapists treat. Children who come in for feeding therapy have developed an aversion to foods for one or more of thousands of reasons. No child with any specific diagnosis is exempt from difficulties with feeding. It is the goal of the OT to help your child to eat safely and in a socially acceptable manner. The OT's role in the feeding team is to work on self-feeding skills. There are times when your child should use his fingers to eat, such as with a sandwich, and times when a fork/spoon is appropriate. The therapist will look at your child's readiness to eat. This means observing his posture, positioning during feeding, his eye/hand coordination, motor skills, and sensory processing skills.

Feeding therapy takes a great deal of time and patience from you, your OT, and your child. A trusting relationship must first be established between the treatment team members, and follow-through with activities from the clinic to home settings is crucial to successful results. If your OT had a miracle cure for picky eaters, millions of parents around the world would be ecstatic! Unfortunately, I have no miracle for you but hope to help you understand why your child is not eating the way you'd like her to. I have spent a great deal of time in my personal life with both of my children in feeding therapy. I can tell you that I understand your frustration and that there IS hope for your child!

What does food aversion mean?

Food aversion is simply the dislike of eating foods with certain textures, colors, smells, or other characteristics determined by the one eating the food. In other words, there is some reason why your child is avoiding a food. Your OT is committed to helping determine exactly what the specific reason or reasons are for the dislike and strong reaction to food. Here's an example:

> Billy is a calm child who listens well to his parents and teachers. He enjoys a wide variety of activities and has friends, but doesn't like getting dirty or wet. In fact, last week there was a rain storm after school and he refused to come out to the carpool until the rain had stopped completely. He has a supportive family that enjoys time spent together. The family tries

each day to sit down to a meal together, but the mealtime usually ends with both Billy and his mom in tears. In fact, mom dreads cooking for the family because she has no idea what Billy's reaction will be to the foods she is preparing. A typical dinnertime begins with Billy fighting not to sit at the table. Mom tries to encourage him with a special toy and other bribes but Billy is still reluctant. After 15 minutes of struggling, Billy sits down but is already agitated. Dinner is cold and the family is feeling anxious. Billy begins to gag at the sight of dad's beans (insert any food that your child is averse to). He also won't take any bites of his own food. He is frustrated that he doesn't get to eat his favorite food, plain noodles, every day. Thirty more minutes pass before the power struggle ends and Billy has eaten none of his dinner. This situation repeats itself at every meal—every day.

If you live with or know a child like Billy, then you know the frustration that can surround mealtime.

Why does my child eat only one or two foods?

We all have foods that are our favorites, but we are willing to try different foods and even variations of that food. Our children are not. They may insist on the same pizza from the same restaurant and if that pizza comes out burned—forget it. I once made pasta for my son and used a new pot. He refused to eat the pasta. It came from the same box and was the same shape as always. He noticed that the pot was different and therefore assumed that the pasta would taste different. Since I had recycled the old pot, we had a serious problem. The pasta standoff lasted over a week until he finally ate a bowl with success.

The key to understanding feeding aversion is to understand it in yourself. Have you ever eaten too much of a food and vomited? You didn't want to eat that food again for a long time. What if you had a stomach virus and vomited up a specific food? For a long time the sight, smell, and taste of that food may cause a reaction in your entire body. You may gag, sweat, or even have to leave the room when you are near that food. It is because of a bad experience that you have formed an opinion. Humans learn based on experience and if the experience is a good one, it's repeated. If it's a bad one, we try to avoid it in the future. Our children may assume that all food may taste like metal if they are using a metal fork. Maybe a detergent used to wash the dishes wasn't rinsed fully and your child remembers the specific taste. They may guess that all plastic plates will make the food "taste funny" and will refuse anything that comes near plastic utensils or plates. One of my clients once choked on a pretzel. He refused any crunchy foods for years because of the one bad experience he had. The problem is compounded when our children have a speech delay and cannot communicate their reasons for not eating. They may not even know what the reasons are. It is the job of the parent and therapist to team up and problem-solve. Additional information on addressing sensory defensiveness in a child's mouth is found in Chapter 5.

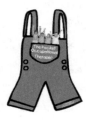

Out of the POCKET Activity

Make a list with two columns. The first one should be what your child currently eats, the second what he used to eat, the third what you'd like for him to eat. Look at the list of current foods and try to note a pattern. For instance, are the foods crunchy or are they mushy? Are the foods sweet, spicy, or sour? Are the foods finger foods or are they fork/spoon foods? Give the list to your OT to help with this analysis.

When you are introducing a new food, encourage your child to play with it first with NO PRESSURE to eat it. Make the activity something at the table with toys, and even place figurines or dolls in the play and pretend to feed the dolls. Do not be discouraged if your child is reluctant to touch the food. In this case, place the food into a plastic bag, seal it, and trace shapes or letters with your fingers on top of the bag onto the food.

Never force your child by holding their hands or feet down in any way while working on feeding. This will be detrimental to him and will erase any progress you've made with him. He must trust you.

How can I tell if my child is having difficulty with eating?

Some signs of eating problems are:

- Coughing, gagging, or choking during eating, playing, or smelling food.

- Needing increased time to eat or complete a meal.

- Eating a limited variety of food.

- Medical issues such as GERD (gastroesophageal reflux disease), reflux, or needing a feeding tube.

- Spitting up food during eating or difficulty keeping liquids in the mouth.

- Difficulty with drinking from an open cup, bottle, or straw.

- Anxiety surrounding eating or preparation of food.

I am a firm believer that a child will succeed if given the chance. As therapists, we need to be vigilant about watching our clients for signs of anxiety and monitor the feeding therapy very closely. When I was a brand new therapist at a feeding clinic, we generally only treated a child as having "behaviors" surrounding eating. We did not look at the problems that may have caused the feeding problems; we solely addressed the behaviors. For instance, one of our children, Tommy, was attending therapy twice per week. His mother wanted him to work on eating peanut butter for lunch at school. Every session ended up with Tommy vomiting and then helping us to clean up the area. During a team meeting, we suggested that maybe something more was going on with Tommy other than a difficulty tolerating the texture. We suggested he see a gastroenterologist and allergist. Dad agreed, and after further testing it was determined that Tommy had a mild allergy to peanuts. We had been trying to work on eating the very food that he was allergic to.

Who should be involved in the "feeding team"?

A team working together to provide support to your child will increase successful outcomes and will help in providing support in a stressful situation. Parents with children who have difficulty with feeding are often stressed and frustrated. They may have feelings of inadequacy and worry that they are being judged by others around them for their child's difficulty. As a parent I understand that frustration and need to connect with others who are going through the same experiences as me. I found that the therapy waiting room was often my favorite place to be as there I felt the camaraderie of other parents who experienced the same feelings as I did.

Often, the OT works together with speech pathologists, physical therapists, dieticians, social workers, case managers, gastroenterologists, allergists, surgeons, and developmental pediatricians. Testing that may be suggested includes:

- Allergy testing to foods that cause vomiting, hives, or asthma. Testing may include skin prick testing where the food or extracts of the suspect food are scratched on the skin. The allergist looks for hives and redness at the site of each prick. RAST (radioallergosorbent) testing is a type of blood test that is used to determine allergies.

- Gastroenterologists (GI) may complete specific swallowing studies such as a videofluorographic swallowing study, which looks at the mechanics of swallowing, if choking or aspiration is suspected; pH probes which look for acidity that can cause reflux; barium swallow which looks at the structure of the pharynx and esophagus; and an EGD or esophagogastroduodenoscopy which is a procedure under sedation where a special scope is used to visualize the esophagus, stomach, and upper intestines.

There are also conditions that may cause feeding difficulty such as cerebral palsy, dysphagia, cleft palate, and stroke, among many others.

Why do sweet, sour, and salty foods matter? What is the texture of a food?

The texture and flavor of a food can be key to whether your child will eat the food or not. It is important to know the differences in order to help to see what your child's preferences are. What do you like to eat? My favorite snack is salty potato chips. I like the way the chips crunch and do not like them when they are stale. The salt is calming to me and when I am having a bad day I often munch on a bag of chips for comfort. There are different levels to texture and flavor. The list below is what *generally* happens with a specific taste, temperature, and texture, although of course, everyone is different:

- *Spicy foods* wake up the senses.

- *Sour foods* increase saliva, causing your oral muscles to work harder to keep the saliva in your mouth.

- *Salty foods* can be calming to some people. Some examples are popcorn and pretzels.

- *Sweet foods* are generally calming to your senses. Candy, sweet juices, hard candies, and pudding are some foods that can be comforting.

- *Cold temperatures* are alerting. People often chew on ice chips to wake them up during a boring seminar.

- *Warm foods* are calming and comforting. Think of a bowl of warm soup on a cold day.

Textures of foods vary from soft to very hard. Texture begins with liquids, then moves on to purees (smooth and lumpy), mushy, firm, crunchy, and mixed. Baby food begins with liquid formula and progresses to stage one smooth foods. As a baby's oral skills develop, he is better able to handle thicker and harder textures. When teeth come in, chewing, biting, and mashing develop and a wide variety of textures is generally accepted. At the same time that the progression of textures from liquid to solids increases, the baby's gag reflex decreases so that he can swallow larger pieces of food.

A hard texture requires more work for chewing so it is generally calming since you are using more mouth muscles. Some people chew on gum to calm them down in a stressful situation.

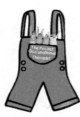

Out of the POCKET Activity

To determine what tastes and textures you prefer, keep a journal for five days. Note the time of day you eat and what taste, texture, and feeling during eating you notice.

- Do you prefer salty snacks at night and are they calming to you?

- When do you need to chew gum or bite into something hard such as a pretzel stick or licorice?

- Do sweet textures bring you relief from stress?

- Do you chew on your pen?

- Are you a person who whistles?

- Do you prefer hot or cold beverages?

- Do you bite your nails?

- Do you eat hard candy during the day?

Now, do the same for your child. Try to note his preferences in taste and texture.

Ask his teacher about his behavior at school. Does he chew on his pencil or place inappropriate items into his mouth? Make sure to note sweet, sour, spicy, or salty. Don't forget about documenting soft, lumpy, or hard. Some children must dip food into a condiment such as ketchup or barbecue sauce. This is important to write down. You may notice a pattern that may help you and your OT to determine a direction to move toward in feeding therapy.

Someone told me that I have to force-feed my child. Is that true?

I am hoping you can learn from my experience.

When my son was two, we attended feeding therapy at a new clinic. The therapist played with him and completed warm-up activities. When he was distracted, she quickly forced him into the high chair, strapped him into it, and placed the tray in front of him. There were three "cues" given to take a bite:

1. "Take a bite."

2. "Take a bite."

3. "Take a bite or I will help you."

He did not bite the food on the third cue, so she held down his hands and forced the spoon into his mouth. He turned his cheek and then she held his head firmly.

I was upset and voiced my displeasure with her therapy. She assured me that this was how therapy was done at the location and after a few weeks he would "come around." I didn't want to be a non-compliant parent and was quite desperate to get him to eat so I agreed to try this technique at home. Feeding only got worse and my son and I were both more frustrated with the process than before we had begun.

Caregivers, trust your gut feeling. Do not permit anyone to force any food or feeding utensil into your child's mouth. Your child will not want to participate in therapy and feeding will get worse.

Thanks to more awareness of feeding therapy and less emphasis on force-feeding, most OTs do not utilize a strictly behavioral approach to feeding. There is a greater push to investigate the reasons for not wanting to eat and the sensory issues involved in feeding. Your OT should use positive behavioral techniques for feeding therapy. Encouragement should be given if your child doesn't spit out the food, if he takes bigger bites, if he doesn't gag when eating a new food, or if he eats a new food independently. Sticker charts, activity rewards, and positive encouragement go a long way with children!

Is it true that you have to exercise mouth/oral muscles before eating?

It is important to "warm up" our muscles before we do hard work. The same is true with our oral musculature.

Children with oral muscle weakness need activities to work their muscles to make them stronger. The masseter or jaw muscle is considered by most to be one of the strongest muscles in your body relative to its small size.

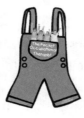

Out of the POCKET Activity

You can feel the masseter. Place your hands on your cheeks. Now, close your mouth and put your back top and bottom teeth together and squeeze them. The masseter is the muscle you feel tightening in your cheek.

Your OT may use tools to warm the muscles up for the "work" of eating. She may use a washcloth to massage the muscles and provide stimulation for the mouth and cheeks. A tool such as a vibratory massager may be rubbed on the inside of the cheeks, tongue, and lips. A fun way to work the tongue is to put something sticky such as peanut butter on your child's lips, and ask her to use her tongue to lick it off! This can be done in front of a mirror for more fun! Use chocolate syrup, whipped cream, or any sticky food your child enjoys. Since this activity is hard work, you may see her drool or become fatigued. Provide lots of praise and encouragement for her! Try to do this activity with her and race for more fun.

Why does my older child drool?

Babies often drool because their oral muscles have not yet developed enough to contain their saliva. Often, babies and younger children drool when they are placed on their tummies and are working their arm, trunk, and leg muscles against gravity. Since the larger muscle groups are working so hard, it is more difficult to gain control over those smaller muscle groups in the mouth. If children have not had the opportunity to strengthen their oral muscles, they won't be able to hold in saliva adequately. Sometimes, the child is not able to feel the drool coming out of his mouth.

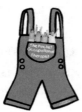 ## Out of the POCKET Activity

For children who are drooling, it is important to increase oral-motor strength and tone in the mouth.

Some children need a cue given to them when they are drooling or placing inappropriate objects into their mouth. The cue can be visual, or placing your finger on the lip so that your child may look at you and know to wipe his mouth. Also, when stimulation is needed to the oral area, a special box can be provided full of fun toys and activities. This box should only be brought out to work on oral-motor activities. A shoe-sized plastic box with small holes punched into it works well. Objects such as whistles, straws, Chewelry (www.kidcompanions.com), Jigglers, and vibratory toys such as those sold in pediatric therapy catalogues should be in the box.

Other ideas for drooling include use of a towel or a vibrating tool to provide massage. Therapists may use ice and soft brushes to provide stimulation to the cheeks and mouth.

How do I help my child to strengthen her mouth/oral muscles?

There are children who have not had enough practice using their mouths for feeding and oral exploration, such as children with feeding tubes and those who have difficulty bringing toys to their mouths due to paralysis, tone, or weakness. These children simply have oral-motor weakness because they have not been given a chance to strengthen their muscles. Remember, all muscles need exercise to keep strong. It is through the therapist's knowledge that this oral muscle weakness is identified and helped with exercises specifically designed for the mouth.

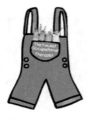

Out of the POCKET Activity

When working with your child on oral muscle exercises, it is important to provide a successful experience every time. So, begin with something easier and every time you work with her, increase the challenge. Try drinking out of a larger straw to start. Make sure the same straws are used by your entire family during dinner. The straw you use should become smaller in size gradually. For example, many fast foods give straws for milkshakes which are larger in diameter. Start with those and then move down to a standard straw which is usually purchased from your local supermarket. Work to drinking from a coffee stirrer. Curly straws of various designs make for hard work too! Try using differently shaped straws.

- Another fun activity is blowing cotton balls through a straw over the table's edge or onto a target.

- Eating popsicles, licorice, gummy worms, chewing gum, and other chewy snacks work the muscles of the mouth.

- Place a mirror in front of your child and then put peanut butter or icing on her lips and ask her to use her tongue to lick it off.

- Tubes of yogurt are good for using muscles to suck the snack out.

- Any whistle, balloon, or activity where your child blows works well.

- One of my favorite activities with clients is placing some non-toxic bubble bath into a plastic shoe-box-sized bin. Fill three-quarters full with water and have your child blow into the water to watch the bubbles pop up. This is fun to try with different colored and scented bubbles.

- Drink thicker liquids such as milkshakes through a smaller straw.

- Cut up vegetables and eat crunchy snacks.

- Try spicy snacks.

- Try a carbonated drink, even carbonated water if you do not allow soda.

Why isn't my child chewing his food?

Some children with decreased muscle strength or decreased tone have difficulty chewing food. We have a refined ability to chew by doing more than moving the jaws up and down. We can also "rotary chew," which means that our jaws are free to move about in a circular motion. Some children need help from an OT to learn how to move their mouths when eating. You may see your OT use a flexible brush (such as a Nuk brush) to place pureed foods on the molars (back teeth) to work on chewing. The tongue also plays a critical part in eating. One of its jobs is to move food around the mouth to ensure it is chewed. The tongue is able to move in all directions to assist in forming sounds when speaking and in moving food around the mouth during feeding. Occupational therapists may use flavor, temperature, and texture as well as other therapeutic tools such as vibration, massage, and having a child eat in front of a mirror to facilitate skills involved with eating.

What does my child's positioning have to do with her eating?

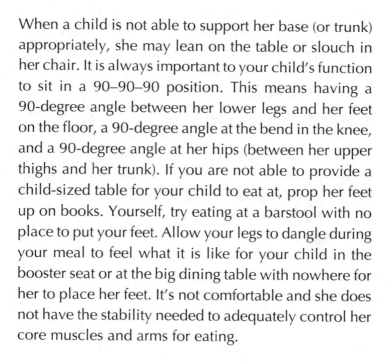

Out of the POCKET Activity

When a child is not able to support her base (or trunk) appropriately, she may lean on the table or slouch in her chair. It is always important to your child's function to sit in a 90–90–90 position. This means having a 90-degree angle between her lower legs and her feet on the floor, a 90-degree angle at the bend in the knee, and a 90-degree angle at her hips (between her upper thighs and her trunk). If you are not able to provide a child-sized table for your child to eat at, prop her feet up on books. Yourself, try eating at a barstool with no place to put your feet. Allow your legs to dangle during your meal to feel what it is like for your child in the booster seat or at the big dining table with nowhere for her to place her feet. It's not comfortable and she does not have the stability needed to adequately control her core muscles and arms for eating.

What does touching different textures with the hands have to do with eating?

Your child with feeding difficulty may exhibit difficulty with getting his hands wet or sticky, or with touching items such as sand or dirt. Often, children demonstrate their aversions to various textures with both hands and mouth. For instance, many children have a great deal of anxiety when their hands get paint or marker on them. Some even gag when their hands get dirty. The child may insist on washing his hands immediately, scrubbing until there is no trace of the mark. Children may also show aversion to getting their hands sticky or touching their food during mealtimes. They prefer use of a utensil even when it seems illogical to use one. One of my clients insisted on using a fork when eating apple slices and a grilled cheese sandwich. She reported that she did not like the feeling of the "slime" on her hands. There are also children who prefer to eat with just one hand since it is too overwhelming to get both hands messy at the same time. Your OT will ask you to list those items that your child will touch and those she won't.

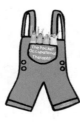

Out of the POCKET Activity

When working with your child on the tolerance of textures on his hands, it is important to begin with a texture that your child is comfortable touching without anxiety. The tactile, or touch, system is the target area. Signs of anxiety are: refusal to touch, gagging when touching different textures, reluctance to participate in an activity using the texture (such as paint) at school, and a tantrum that comes seemingly from nowhere when presented with the item.

- To begin, start with a dry texture. Rice, leaves, and raw beans are examples. Place the items in a plastic bin along with some other items such as paper clips, toy cars, or blocks. Ask your child to search through the box to find different items. Your child should be comfortable with this activity for at least three play sessions without signs of anxiety before moving on.

- The next texture in sequence is an in-between texture, such as play dough, cooked pasta, or sand. Your child should be able to play comfortably in these items without immediately washing his hands or gagging. Make play fun!

- Finally, introduce messy and slimy play with wet paint, pudding, or yogurt, for example. If your child isn't ready for direct contact with the materials, place them into a plastic bag and seal it. Encourage your child to trace letters on top of the bag first until she is comfortable. Place fun toys into the bin with the slime and do not draw attention to the mess. It can be difficult for some parents to have "messy play" in their home. Designate an area, preferably at the dinner table, to help the child to be comfortable in the meal area.

Ways to work on holding feeding utensils and scooping up food

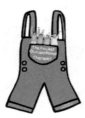 ## Out of the POCKET Activity

The best way to work on eating skills is to practice in a fun way. Use dough to make hot dogs or pizzas and then cut them with a plastic or butter knife. Your child can play with his toys and pretend to have a party with food.

Make play cakes and slice pieces up for the guests. My clients used to love working with wooden 3-D food puzzles, with pizzas, vegetables, and loaves of bread held together by Velcro and with a wooden knife to cut the items up into pre-sliced pieces. This is a fun way to work on eating in a play setting.

Fill a bin with rice and beans and use spoons to scoop them up into different containers. Sand boxes could hold spoons of various sizes and colors to play with. Scooping water with different-sized scoops is fun and good for summertime play!

Why is my child making so many "odd" noises with his mouth?

Children who make noises such as clicking, teeth grinding, humming, and high pitched noises may actually find that making the noises is calming. Some kids enjoy the feeling of tightening the muscles of the mouth, body, tongue, neck, and vocal cords. However, others around your child may be distracted by the noise.

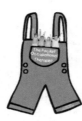

Out of the POCKET Activities

- Provide oral-motor toys such as Chewigems, Z-Vibes, Chewlery.

- Allow your child to drink from a coffee stirrer as it gives work to the oral musculature.

- Practice massage of the cheek muscles.

- Place a small amount of whipped cream on the lips and encourage use of the tongue to lick off the cream. This activity forces the tongue to work.

- Allow your child to use noise-cancelling headphones to block out any possible loud noises in the environment.

- Provide relaxing music via headphones to comfort your child.

What if my child is never hungry OR never seems to be full?

Our body receives information from the organs. This information helps us to feel hunger, thirst, bowel and bladder sensations, and nausea, among many others. The brain receives information from the receptors and cues the body to regulate breathing, heart rate, contractions of the bladder, and those necessary adjustments needed to keep your body alive. Interoception is a sense that gives us information about our internal body. Through it, we receive sensations of hunger, our heart rate, pain, and thirst, among many others. When your body needs food, your stomach tells the brain that it's hungry. However, if a child has difficulty processing sensory information (see Chapter 5), he may not "feel" or register the feelings of hunger.

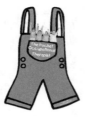

Out of the POCKET Activities

- Keep your child on a sensory diet. It's not a food diet but an activity diet to help to regulate the sensory system. Heavy work involving pushing, pulling, lifting, and carrying should be completed on a regular basis of at least every two hours.

- Use your child's favorite scents to help bring on hunger. What flavors does your child prefer? Use scented oils, markers or Smencils pencils to stimulate appetite. For example, when my younger son smells chocolate, he gets hungry. Remember that receptors in our nose are very closely linked to our feelings area of the brain. Smell can be extremely powerful to evoke emotions. Think about some of your favorite holidays and the smell of food cooking!

- Encourage SMALL bites for children who overeat or stuff their mouths.

- Use a bite chart. After EACH bite, allow your child to place a sticker on a chart. The act of putting down the fork gives the child time to clear his mouth.

- Ask your child to eat one bite and then drink a sip of liquid. Again, the liquid will help to clear food from the mouth.

- Give small portions.

- Encourage children to blow bubbles, cotton balls or ping pong balls with straws. Heavy work of the mouth often helps to "warm up" muscles involved with eating.

Chapter 4

Handwriting and the Upper Extremity (Arm)

What are fine motor skills?

Fine motor skills involve the use of our arms, hands, and fingers. The skills begin to develop at birth and are critical in the use of the hands to grasp and manipulate objects such as writing and feeding utensils, scissoring, and items for self-care. We have 27 bones and 38 muscles which help to move our hands. Our body generally follows a predictable pattern of development. Gross motor skills are the use of large muscle groups for movements of the entire body. Walking, running, crawling, sitting upright, and rolling are activities that utilize these large muscle groups. It is important to remember that the acquisition of gross motor skills directly affects the ability to perform most fine motor skills. Our bodies generally develop head to toe (cephalo to caudal) and center of the body to the sides (or proximal to distal).

How do grasp and hand use develop?

The process of hand development begins in infancy. When a baby is born, he can grasp your finger reflexively. By four months he is beginning to bat at his toys with one or both arms. His hands can grasp large items such as his bottle and blocks with all or most fingers.[1] He is not able to release objects yet as the grasp is still reflexive. Soon his body begins to work against gravity and more purposeful body movements develop. One of the key ingredients to developing hand coordination is weight bearing through his arms. As he begins to crawl and move, his mobility depends on both arms and legs. It is important to remember that development of many other body systems are important in relation to the hands. The baby must also be able to visualize, feel, and turn toward the item he is attempting to grasp.

What are intrinsic muscles?
What is "in-hand" manipulation?

Many children with weakness of the hand musculature have difficulty developing a tripod grasp. Some children are simply developing at a slower pace than others and the grasp develops later on. One of the biggest issues that occupational therapists help our clients with is weakness in the hands for buttoning, tying, and handwriting. There are many muscles that

---

1   Buckland, D. J., Edwards, S. J. and McCoy-Powlen, J. D. (2002) *Developmental and Functional Hand Grasps.* Thorofare, NJ: Slack Inc.

begin in the forearm and end in the hand which flex and extend the fingers. It is important to note that there are also muscles that originate inside the hand called intrinsic muscles. They are responsible for intricate movements (dexterity) of the fingers and thumb. A skill called translation is when a small object is moved from the palm to the fingertips and back again. The fingers also are capable of rotating an object at the fingertips. Often, the intrinsic muscles are weak and must be strengthened in order to complete buttoning, tying, and scissoring activities.

In-hand manipulation is the ability to use both sides of the hand for completion of a task. So, the hand must be able to complete two movements at the same time. For example, write with a pencil and then turn it so that the eraser side is toward the paper, keeping the pencil in the same hand. Do not help with the other hand! Your fingers are able to work together with the palm of your hand to move the pencil.

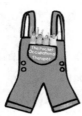 ## Out of the POCKET Activity

Place a pile of pennies on the table. Pick one up with your dominant hand (the hand you write with) and move the penny to your palm without the help of your other hand. Now, use your ring and pinky fingers to hold the penny you've just picked up while trying with your thumb and pointer finger to pick up more pennies. Don't let go of the pennies you picked up. Try to hold them in your palm. You will feel the intrinsic hand muscles working hard during this task involving *translation*.

How can I help my child to button, zip, and snap? Why is my child not able to use a tripod grasp?

Your child may be using a stable grasp. This means that she may be using all of the muscles that she can to stabilize her hand while writing due to weak muscles. She may be placing all of her fingers on the pencil. When a muscle or group of muscles is weak, our bodies use a strategy called "compensation." Compensation means that we try to use other muscles or different movements to make up for a weakness.

It is key to make sure that her feet are flat on the floor and she is not sitting in a chair that's too big or too small for her. She should be sitting at a 90–90–90 position when doing any handwriting or scissoring. If her feet aren't flat on the floor, use a stool or old phone book to place under her feet. (See the section in Chapter 2 under "What does positioning mean?" for details.)

It is important to encourage fun activities which are strategically designed to work on strengthening her thumb, pointer, and middle finger. The more practice she has using them together, the better able she will be to complete a tripod grasp.

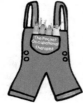

Out of the POCKET Activities

- Break her crayons in half so that she has a smaller surface area on which to place her fingers. Use a golf pencil with an eraser placed on top as a smaller pencil.

- Encourage her to work with putty or dough to find small craft beads or coins.

- Cut a slit into the top of a cream cheese container. Have her place small items into the slit, such as colored paper clips, coins, and small pegs.

- Tear small pieces of tissue paper up and use fingers to roll them up and glue them onto a piece of construction paper to make patterns.

- Use tweezers to pick small items up. Therapy catalogues have fun colored and shaped tweezers that children love.

- Use an inclined surface while writing and doing crafts. A chalk or white board that can incline is a super idea for writing on. A child is much more likely to use the proper wrist and hand motions while using an angled surface to work on.

- Use a three-ring binder that is four inches wide. Place the paper on a clipboard on top of the binder. The use of the binder provides an inclined surface which helps with positioning of the hand and wrist for handwriting.

- Use an eye dropper to transfer water from one container to another. It's fun if you use food coloring or glitter to make the water bright.

- Use small stampers of different shapes. It's fun to correlate the stamps with an upcoming holiday. Sometimes, stores carry stampers for a low price around the season or holiday.

- Perler beads come in all different colors. Picking up such a small bead is wonderful for developing fine motor skills.

Is it OK to use grippers on my child's pencil?

Occupational therapists have varying opinions on the issue of gripper use. It is generally accepted that if the gripper is too hard or too large, it will most likely be uncomfortable. Grippers that are small and soft are good choices. Experiment with several types on your own pencil with your child to see what works best for each of you. Some children have a grip that is too loose, while some grippers allow extra large areas for easier grasp. Ask your child's teacher or school OT if any grippers have been used in the classroom.

What can I do to help my child to develop hand dominance?

It is important that your child develop a preference for one hand as the dominant one as he enters school. This means that you will notice that one of your child's hands will be the "leader" and one will be the "helper." There are many activities you can do at home to work on development of a dominant hand. Make sure to work slowly over time and ensure your child has fun while completing the activities. Remember that a child's work is his play, and it is through play that he learns valuable skills.

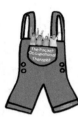

Out of the POCKET Activities

Remember to look for the hand that is faster and more skilled when completing the following activities. If your child's stronger hand gets tired, ask her to rest and not to switch hands for the activity. She will need time to build up her muscles—as with any exercise.

- Work with tools such as hammering pegs or screwing in large bolts.

- Open and close/screw and unscrew lids onto containers of various sizes. The more skilled hand will better be able to open the lids and the helper hand will be the one stabilizing the container.

- Work on mazes and tracing activities. The dominant hand will hold the pencil and the helper will stabilize the paper.

- Scoop sand into different containers. Make scoops of different sizes and colors for fun.

- Pour liquid from one container into another. My clients like it when I use food coloring to make the water change colors when they pour them into one another.

- Use a turkey baster to transfer water from one container into another one. The dominant hand will be the one the child uses to squeeze the baster and the helper will hold the container to stabilize it.

- There are wonderful wooden puzzles that work on pretend cutting. There are fruits, vegetables, and loaves of bread held together by Velcro. Children love these puzzles and they also encourage pretend play.

How can I work on cutting/scissoring skills with my child?

Scissoring skills are great for children to learn since so many fun activities involve this skill. Many kindergartens expect your child to be proficient in scissors use. The strong emphasis on hands-on learning is a wonderful thing in today's classroom, but when a child is weak in scissors use, he may become frustrated and lag behind the class during center times (individual or small-group activities).

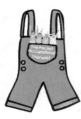

Out of the POCKET Activity

Learning how to hold the scissors correctly requires practice. Begin by working with your child on the concept of opening/releasing. The use of tongs to squeeze and release items of various sizes is excellent practice. You can use regular tongs or order ones of all shapes and sizes from therapy catalogues listed in the resource section at the end of this book. Turkey basters or small droppers are fun ways to encourage squeeze and release. Color the water with food coloring for more fun. Use hole punchers of all shapes and sizes. Clothes pins can be clipped onto the edge of shoe boxes to make patterns. Note how your child is using both of his hands together as one should be completing the activity and the other should be the helper (see next section for more details). Scissoring is a skill where one hand holds the tool and the other is responsible for moving the paper in different directions.

Begin with the actual scissors and ask your child to snip the paper to make "grass" or "hair." Next, have your child cut across narrow strips of paper so that he can see that he's actually cut through the entire thing. Cut strips of paper of different colors and glue together to make a paper chain. To start with, have your child make shapes by cutting along thick and straight lines. Then gradually make the lines wavy and then progress to different shapes and sizes. Make sure he is successful and provide lots of encouragement. It takes time to build up those hand muscles and just like everything else we do, practice is so important.

Note: If your child is left-handed, please purchase the correct scissors for left-handed children. It will definitely make the task easier if he has the proper tools. Encourage the school to provide him with the scissors or purchase them on your own and make sure they stay in his pencil box for center time.

What is bilateral integration?

Bilateral means both sides, and integration is working together. So, bilateral integration is when both sides of the body work together to complete a task. Often, the hands are completing different tasks to accomplish a common goal. There is awareness of both sides, right and left. Generally, one side is dominant or the one actually completing the job and the other is used as a stabilizer. When a child has difficulty in this area, she may avoid crossing her midline. This means that she may not be able to coordinate her hands together to complete a task. For example, she may have difficulty with scissoring since it requires one hand to cut while the other stabilizes the paper. A child with poor bilateral integration may also have trouble with lacing shoes, jumping jacks, bicycle riding, and threading beads. Sometimes a child may appear "clumsy" and may have a great deal of frustration. Many of my clients have difficulty cutting meat with a fork and knife. This task requires both hands to work together.

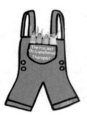 ## Out of the POCKET Activities

Children with bilateral integration difficulty should be given motivating tasks that are specifically planned to be fun:

- The use of a rolling pin requires both hands. Set up a bakery and use the hands together to roll, pat, and create pastries out of real or play dough.

- Shuffle cards and play card games which require the child to hold the cards in one hand and pick up with the other.

- Provide containers of different sizes to practice opening and closing. Place a treat in each one for a fun surprise!

- String beads of different shapes and sizes.

- Begin to work on shoe tying by using lacing boards or cards with holes punched in them.

- Squeeze sponges of different shapes. Use colored water for more fun.

- Play hide and seek with various shaped items in putty or dough.

- Tearing paper is a fun activity to do with smaller children. Use your paper to make a craft. Squeezing a large container of glue with both hands adds an extra challenge.

- Fold socks, towels, and other laundry.

- Set up a t-ball area in your yard or garden and use arms to swing at the ball.

What does it mean to cross the midline?

A midline is an imaginary line in the middle of the body. When we are babies, we learn to bring our hands together and reach for toys with our hands while sitting on the floor. The ability for your child to cross her midline is extremely important for developing motor skills. It goes hand in hand with bilateral integration. As we develop, one of our hands becomes the dominant one and the other is the helper. If we do not develop a dominant hand, we do not refine the skills of either hand for writing, dressing, eating, and scissoring. When we read a page, our eyes must scan across the entire page. During writing, a child should be able to draw a horizontal line across the entire page with one hand and not switch hands in the middle. Many children prefer to use their right hand for activities on the right side of their body and their left hand for things on the left side of their body.

Many of my clients demonstrate the lack of ability to cross their midline. Here's an example. Your daughter is working on a puzzle. You notice that she spreads all of the pieces of the puzzle onto the table. She uses her right hand to pick up and place the pieces on the right side of the table and her left hand to pick up and place the pieces on the left side of the table. When you ask her to pick up a piece of the puzzle on the left side of the table with her right hand, she turns her entire body (trunk). It sounds confusing, but once you understand what crossing the midline means, you will see how important the skill is for a lifetime of success in activities of daily living.

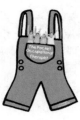

Out of the POCKET Activities

You may need to provide encouragement for your child to cross his hands across his body. Have fun with the activities listed below and be sure to ask your child not to move his body (trunk) side to side, but instead have his arms move to cross the imaginary line across the center of his body.

- Play games of pat-a-cake. Encourage your child to hit your right hand with his right, and your left hand with his left.

- Use a large poster board or butcher paper and fill it with shapes and colors.

- Place the child on his tummy and play a board game or work a puzzle. This will require him to cross over the board to move and arrange the pieces.

- Stand next to your child and pass a basketball back and forth. Put on some music and make a chain of friends and pass the ball in one direction. Switch directions when you stop the music.

- Sit back to back and pass a ball around your body to each other. My clients love doing this to fun, bouncy music.

- Scrub down a chalkboard or use a sponge to clean large windows together. Hold the sponge or brush with both hands.

- Work on paper/pencil activities such as matching the doggie to his bone. Draw the doggie on the left side of the paper and the bone on the right side of the paper. Make sure your child doesn't move the paper while drawing the line, but instead moves his pencil across the paper. You can draw anything you want that may go together and interests your child. Mazes, word searches, and tracing are other paper/pencil activities you can try.

- Using a large whiteboard or chalkboard, draw a figure eight lying on its side (like the infinity sign). Have your child stand in front of the middle of the shape and trace the shape back and forth. Encourage him to cross his arm across his body while completing the activity.

My child has weak arms. What can we do at home?

An occupational therapist is specially trained to complete testing called Manual Muscle Testing. This series of tests allows the OT to separate out groups of muscles. A number is assigned based on the amount of resistance to gravity and to pressure gently applied to the muscle by the therapist. If your child has difficulty raising her arm against gravity or with lifting something heavy, strengthening activities are designed to target her areas of weakness. Ask your OT which muscles are weak and to suggest activities or a home exercise program. Be sure that your OT demonstrates how to correctly perform the exercises with you and your child. Ask any questions you have and if you are unsure about the correct way to do an exercise, do not do it until you have full understanding of its completion.

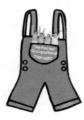

Out of the POCKET Activities

- Hold arms straight out to the sides at shoulder height and move them in small circles ten times forward and ten times backwards.

In the same position, make large circles with the arms ten times forward and then repeat backwards.

- Practice bouncing a basketball. This is a good coordination and strengthening activity.

- Use a large beach ball to play volleyball in the back yard or garden with a friend.

- Animal walking is a fun activity. Ask your child to crawl like a crab on the floor. He can walk like a bear, hop on all fours like a frog, or lie on his belly to pretend to slither on the ground like a snake.

- Wall push-ups are fun if your child pretends that the wall is falling down and he must use his arms positioned at shoulder height to help hold up the wall.

- There are many colored therapy or yoga balls that weigh one or two pounds. Ask older children to slowly raise their arms in front of them and then slowly lower them. Repeat ten times. Smaller children may enjoy gently tossing the weighted balls into a target such as a hula hoop.

Chapter 5

What Do You Mean, We Have More Than Five Senses?

What are the other senses?

Each of us knows that there are five senses: vision (visual), hearing (auditory), smell (olfactory), oral (gustatory), and touch (tactile). There have been huge advances in our understanding of the way our bodies obtain and process sensory information and most OTs have a good knowledge of this. If you are told that your child has sensory processing disorder or difficulty with sensory integration and needs OT treatment, make sure to ask your therapist about his/her training and experience with clients with sensory processing disorder. If the OT doesn't know that there are more than five senses, ask for another therapist.

Let's review the obvious senses to ensure a full understanding of the sensory system:

- VISION (VISUAL): The ability to see color, physical properties, and pattern as well as the ability to utilize the eye muscles to focus, track a moving object, and discriminate (receive and interpret information about our environment) are all components of vision. Visual perception involves the body's ability to decipher relationships about people and objects in our environment. Perception includes the memory and experiences we have had in the past. Visual perception helps us to detect differences in things we see such as physical traits and specific details.

- HEARING (AUDITORY): The ability to respond to and interpret sound, vibration, and movement. The inner ear contains the receptors for sound. Processing of sounds that we receive is important to determine their meaning. For example, a high-pitched sound such as a siren is generally alerting to us. High-pitched sounds give us details about the location of sound. When we hear a sound that is familiar or comforting, such as our mother's voice, we react or feel certain emotions. So, auditory information actually involves receiving or hearing the sound through receptors in the inner ear and then auditory processing gives "meaning" to the sound after organizing and categorizing it.

- SMELL (OLFACTORY): Our nose contains sensory receptors which send information to the olfactory bulb located in the mid-brain. The interesting fact about smells is that a smell can take a direct "shortcut" to the part of the brain that is responsible for emotional memory—the limbic system. So, smell is unique as it is extremely powerful to our sensory system. What does your favorite food smell like? What odor is your least favorite? Imagine the smell of garbage rotting in an alley on a hot day. Now, imagine the smell of Thanksgiving dinner. The smells we have experienced in our lives directly affect emotions and memories we have formed.

- ORAL (GUSTATORY): The oral system consists of the chemical receptors on the tongue called taste buds, the tongue and cheeks, and the connections to the nervous system which allow us to process taste. Textures of foods are interpreted by the gustatory system. Babies explore the world around them by "mouthing" objects as they develop. In addition, a baby obtains nourishment by suckling on breast or bottle. As he develops, he learns to calm himself down by sucking on his thumb, pacifier, or other object. There are many people who chew their nails, ice, gum or other objects to calm themselves when in a stressful situation or due to anxiety. Oral input is extremely important throughout our lives. If a child has a bad experience or does not like a certain taste, the memory of the experience may cause anxiety surrounding future eating or oral experiences. One of the most important things about the oral area is that the mouth is one of the most sensitive areas and is an extremely personal area of the body. I have heard in two different conferences that attempting to force-feed a child or forcing oral-motor tools may be considered an extreme invasion of personal space and can cause severe anxiety that may not be overcome—even with prolonged therapeutic interventions.

- TOUCH (TACTILE): The tactile system allows us to receive sensation through contact with our skin. Information about temperature, pressure, and pain comes through our tactile system. It is also responsible for alerting us to a hot stove, stepping on glass, or frost-bite. It is a system that is protective and helps us to orient ourselves to our surroundings by letting us know something is touching our body. Information about how much pressure is being applied, where the pressure is, and the size and shape of the object touching us are all detected via the tactile system. Tolerating and interpreting touch and various experiences we have through touch is critical to our early and continued development and learning how to explore our environment. Babies are born with defensive senses for their survival, and as they develop they learn to explore and make sense of how their body relates to the environment, which helps them to master skills. Fine motor skills are extremely dependent on touch as our mouth and hands have more tactile receptors than anywhere else in the human body.

In addition to these five senses, the proprioceptive system and vestibular system are key in our daily functioning:

- PROPRIOCEPTIVE: Proprioception involves movement of our bodies. There are many receptors in our bodies—specifically in our joints, tendons, and muscles—whose job is to perceive movement. Types of movement may be stretching, compression, and bending. The receptors send sensory information about the type of movement, pressure, position, and impact to the central nervous system. This input allows us to locate our body in space. As a result, our body can then plan motor (movement) actions, become aware of where our body is or how is it positioned, and then form an appropriate behavior or response.

  The proprioceptive system develops with the tactile and vestibular systems. Visual input can also influence our knowledge of where our body is in space. When an infant crawls and works her body against gravity by rolling, sitting, and moving in space, her body learns to receive information, process it in the central nervous system, and then form an output or action. The success of coordinating—of having the baby's body work as a whole—depends on the ability to integrate and react to information obtained via proprioception.

• VESTIBULAR: The vestibular system involves the inner ear, which can detect changes in position and movement. Vestibular information gives us information about the speed and direction in which we are moving. The developing fetus is capable of responding to specific movement. This is because gravity is constantly pulling on our body and, as a result, we are always responding to it by changing positions and adapting our body to maintain an upright position for stability. The inner ear passes information through a complex network of connections to the brain. Balance and movement affect our muscle tone, vision, alertness, awareness of our body in space, and even level of fatigue as we struggle to work our body against gravity.

The vestibular system's importance in our daily functioning is best described and understood when we consider the effect an inner ear infection or "head cold" has on our daily activities. We may experience dizziness, nausea/vomiting, headaches, visual disturbances, and auditory (hearing) disturbances which may greatly affect our ability to function. Sometimes, it is even difficult to explain and understand how much anxiety we can have when affected by issues with our vestibular system. You can imagine how difficult it may be for a child with a special need and difficulties with communication to understand and describe how irritating and debilitating dysfunctions in his vestibular system could feel.

What is modulation of our sensory system?

Our existence and success in our daily functioning is dependent directly on the input—or information we receive—through our senses, our processing of that input, and our formulation of the correct output or response. This happens at a subconscious level.

We can think of our body as a computer. The mouse and keyboard put in the information, the processor functions as the brain, and the output is formed. When there is something wrong or there is a "glitch" in any part of the process, there will be some kind of disruption. There are many ways information enters and is perceived by our body and then, based on how we enter in that information and process it according to our unique experiences, we formulate an output or response. Modulation, then, is the balance between our level of arousal and the intensity of the stimulation we are experiencing. We use our body's modulation to respond to the environment. Some equate our internal modulation to a thermostat. The problem comes when someone has sensory processing dysfunction, where the level of response may not fit the level required.

Some people have heightened arousal levels (hyper-sensitive), low arousal levels (hypo-sensitive), or mixed levels. The most important point is that the reactions our body has to the information we receive can affect our heart rate, temperature, sweating, blood vessels, digestion, and so on. How would you react if a snake began crawling up your leg? Some would "freak out" and scream, sweat, cry, and their heart rate would rise. Others may simply reach down and remove the snake without much thought. Some of the response you form depends on your body's interpretation of the feeling of the snake, its sound, the sight of it, and some of your response depends on your past experiences in life.

Everyone exists at a different level of sensory alertness. Whether or not someone has sensory processing disorder, his body needs to be able to receive and process sensory input. Consider a room where there is a business meeting. The temperature of the room is set to 68 degrees F. Some people in the room are perfectly comfortable at this temperature, some are warm, and some are cold. The way the room feels to someone depends on the level at which they receive the temperature. If someone is already stressed due to a difficult morning or running late for the meeting, he may already be over-stimulated and may already have been warm or over-heated prior to entering the meeting. What if someone is extremely tired due to a sleepless night? He may be chilly sitting in the room since his body is existing at a hypo-responsive state. The same room feels totally different to everyone sitting in that room due to prior experience and current state of alertness.

What do we take away from the above scenario? Our existence in the situation we are in right now depends on our experiences prior to this point in time. This is true for every person, and our children with sensory processing disorder are no exception. A child may wake up after a restless night of sleep. He may be agitated and hyper-responsive to noise, the feeling of his clothing as he gets dressed, the feeling of the crunchy, pinchy cereal he's eating for breakfast, the noise of the school bus as the children talk on the way to school. He is already operating at a heightened level of alertness and he is hyper-responsive. We expect him to sit in his seat quietly and pay attention to hours of classroom instruction. He may exhibit disruptive behaviors as a result of his attempts to organize himself and then have his recess taken away as a punishment. He may tantrum, not due to "bad" or attention-seeking behavior, but due to his frustration. It is our job as parents, teachers, and therapists to play detective and to help our children figure out their general baseline and triggers to sensory overload. We should make lists, charts, and do whatever is necessary to help learn about our children's sensory systems. I guarantee your hard work will pay off!

What does successful sensory processing/integration mean to my child and his abilities?

With successful integration of the input we receive, we formulate an appropriate response to our environment and the situation. When we succeed, we form a memory of the event that should be repeated because it was enjoyable and successful. The ability to overcome a situation or challenge in the environment with a good result means that our body "learns" through practice and then we become more organized in our behaviors. When the brain is organized, we then gain confidence in ourselves and in our ability to function in our world. For example, suppose you are a fan of coffee. You set the timer on your coffee pot and wake up to the smell of the coffee brewing. The smell comes into your body via your olfactory sense. You associate the smell of coffee with a pleasurable experience of relaxation and enjoyment. As you successfully walk toward the kitchen, you maintain your posture, balance, and position against gravity. When you reach out, you accidentally pour the coffee onto your hand instead of into the cup. Reflexively, you interpret the hot coffee as a painful experience and remove your hand. Finally, you pour the coffee into your cup, take a drink, and enjoy the warmth of the coffee in your mouth. You are especially happy because you have added some sweet vanilla creamer, the taste of which you enjoy.

What does sensory processing dysfunction look like in a classroom setting from a child's perspective?

A child who has hyper-sensitivity may be over-aroused and may pay attention to every stimulus around her. She tends to avoid input to her body. Picture her sitting in the classroom during a lesson on geography. She cannot screen out sounds, sights, smells, tactile/touch items which are not appropriate or necessary to process what she needs to...the teacher's voice and the overhead projector. So, what does she experience? The classroom temperature may be too hot, she hears the buzzing of the fluorescent lights, the sniffling of her classmate's running nose due to a cold, the hardness of the chair she's sitting on, the sound of a passer-by in the hallway, the smell of lunch baking in the cafeteria, the feeling of her needing to use the restroom soon, and so on. She may become irritated and agitated with nowhere to place her irritated energy. Her body may feel anxiety where her heartbeat increases, she begins to sweat, and she may even begin to breathe rapidly. If she isn't able to verbalize or take a break from what is happening to her at this moment, she may act out during the next class or begin to move her body in a disruptive way that may interrupt the teacher. It can be a vicious cycle for children who have difficulty integrating their sensory systems.

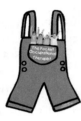

Out of the POCKET Activity

What to look for when considering hyper-sensitivity (over-reaction or reaction with alarm) to sensory input in your child:

- Strong preference for upright postures and delayed balance with possible fear of unexpected movements against gravity.

- Difficulty riding a bicycle.

- Low muscle tone.

- Fear of loud noises or over-reaction to unexpected noises.

- Hyper-sensitivity to smells or tastes.

- Limited repertoire of foods.

- Over-reaction to touch from other children or when accidentally bumped.

- Agitation when standing close to others in line or sitting in a crowded setting such as a cafeteria, concert, or public place.

- Meltdowns during dressing due to tags, seams, or textures.

- Motion/car sickness.

- Difficulty transitioning between summer and winter clothing.

- Agitation during bathing, grooming, teeth brushing, hair combing.

- Poor visual integration—lost in space.

What to look for when considering hypo-sensitivity (under-sensitive or craving/needing more stimulation) in your child:

- May have high pain tolerance such as not noticing a cut or severe bruise. (I had one client who had been bitten by over 20 fire ants and didn't notice the large welts on his body. He stated that he didn't feel anything despite being taken to the ER for treatment of the wounds.)

- Craving movement activities, twirling, spinning, swinging, and jumping constantly during the day.

- Impulsivity and dangerous behaviors such as jumping off high furniture without considering the consequences.

- Difficulty with processing directions and sounds.

- Delays in speech with pronunciation and focusing on foreground sounds.

- Poor coordination during visual tasks.

- Wiggles in seat.

- Enjoys making sounds.

- Prefers loud music.

- Reacts inappropriately to others' feelings.

- Smells objects constantly.

- Mouths objects frequently that aren't food or aren't age-appropriate.

Mixed hypo-hyper frequently occurs and any of the above can occur along with the following:

- Writes too hard/soft with pencil.

- Reacts with anger, sadness, or fear to social situations.

- May avoid interaction in social situations.

- May not consider others' feelings.

- Difficult to calm down.

- Has difficulty with transitioning and completing tasks.

Whether your child is hyper-sensitive, hypo-sensitive, or mixed has the potential to severely impact his ability to function in our world. It is critical to determine which stimuli are pertinent to a certain situation and which aren't. The child with difficulty processing sensory information requires a lot of patience and a strong understanding that the child is not simply acting out for attention. The sensory processing dysfunction is a real issue and can be a huge obstacle to successful completion of activities of daily living.

Why does my child crash into people and furniture all of the time?

A child who demonstrates rough play and frequently crashes his body into items and people may have difficulty with proprioception. Imagine that you are wearing a glove on your hand. Without using your vision, feel around in your purse for your lipstick while wearing that glove. It is difficult to feel the exact shape and size as well as the texture of the lipstick container.

A child with hypo-sensitivity may not be able to get a good feel for what position her body is in. She may need the additional input that crashing gives to fully understand where her body is in space. A child may even get a bump or bruise on her body during rough playing and not even be aware of it. This behavior should be noted by the caregiver to determine things such as what time of day it happens. Does it happen during or after periods of homework or time spent seated for quiet time? The OT will suggest activities such as providing a weighted blanket, hugs, or even tighter clothing to provide her body with additional input to help to regulate her system.

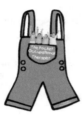

Out of the POCKET Activity

Heavy work is an important intervention for helping with "body in space" issues. Theraband exercises, using a beanbag chair, hugs, swimming, karate, yoga, climbing on playground equipment, playing in the sand, helping with household chores such as vacuuming and lifting groceries are excellent activities. Massage to the arms and legs with lotion is calming. So also is use of vibration such as a Z-Vibe to the mouth, massage to cheeks with a washcloth, and drinking out of a thin straw. Warm baths are a relaxing way to end the day. Any input that is given to the proprioceptive system may last for about one and a half to two hours.

Why is my child chewing on his shirt, pencil, or other items which are not appropriate? Why is my child gagging and stuffing food into his mouth?

A child with sensory processing dysfunction may frequently chew on non-food items or on items not appropriate for his age. Children with a decreased ability to "feel" what is going on inside their mouth may crave additional input to the mouth to help to increase attention or calm themselves down. An infant uses sucking on a pacifier, bottle, or his thumb to calm himself down. As he gets older, he learns other ways of calming that are age-appropriate. Some children may chew on their pencil, clothing, or even their fingers.

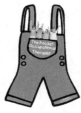

Out of the POCKET Activity

Ways to help older children calm themselves down include chewing bagels or chewy foods, use of straws to blow small pieces of paper off a desk in a race with other children, use of whistles, vibratory input via a Z-Vibe, and massage. In school, a piece of clear tubing may be placed on the end of a child's pencil so that she can safely chew without eating the pencil wood or eraser. Chewing on Chewelry or jewelry children can chew on is a socially acceptable way of getting oral input and stimulation. Also, working on ways to calm herself via heavy work through her entire body and completing regular sensory activities throughout the day will help a child to regulate her system.

Bite charts are a good way to decrease food "stuffing." Encourage your child to take a bite and then move a piece on a game board or place a token on a chart. This will slow her down. Another idea is to take a bite and then a drink afterwards. Make a cue or sign that only you and your child will know, such as placing a finger to your cheek, while out in public to cue her to slow down until she learns on her own. Stuffing can be dangerous as it is a choking hazard. Like all skills, decreasing stuffing takes time, patience, and practice.

Why is my child not getting dressed? Why does my child hate tags and logos on his clothes?

A child with a hyper-responsive system is sensitive to things that many of us may not even notice. Seams on socks or clothing, tags, and pictures or logos on shirts may be perceived by our children differently to how we imagine. Some children describe these feelings as itchy, burning, scraping, painful, or stinging like a bee sting. The challenge comes when we have a child with decreased verbalization or no verbal communication at all. It is our responsibility to figure out what is bothering our children.

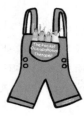

Out of the POCKET Activity

See the resource section at the end of this book for websites specializing in clothing for children with hyper-sensitivity to clothing.

Your OT can help you to make a chart or list of common behaviors or anxieties that happen during the day and will help you to make sense of them. She may help you with a sensory diet or activity diet to help maintain the "just right" or comfortable level of alertness. A therapeutic brushing program can be a helpful tool. The brush has soft bristles and is used directly on the child's skin. The OT will demonstrate the technique on your child and then you must demonstrate proficiency before you try the technique at home. The brushing is done on a schedule and good results may be seen in tolerating dressing and bathing as well as in other daily living areas.

Why is my child dizzy all of the time? Why is my child falling down so much?

Children with difficulty in the vestibular system along with other areas may exhibit difficulty in coordination and balance. You may notice trouble with bicycle riding, hopping, skipping, and other gross or large body movements. Gym class or sports may be difficult or frustrating and other children may even make fun of your child. There are some of us who enjoy riding amusement park rides and some who do not. The variance of tolerance to movement activities is normal from person to person. The same is true for our children.

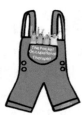

Out of the POCKET Activity

We must begin at a level which is comfortable for our children and then move at a pace that is comfortable and not scary. The unique training of the OT allows her to be proficient at giving children the "just-right" challenge. That means to complete activities where your child is successful to build confidence slowly and then progress very gradually until success is achieved. The use of swings, scooters, inclines (ramps), and balance boards are common in occupational therapy sessions. Tools and activities that look like play are truly designed to be therapeutic. The most important thing to note is to choose an OT who understands the sensory system and how to target the specific areas that each client needs to work on.

There are two types of swinging: *linear*—in a line or front to back such as a tree swing; and *rotary*—in a circular direction such as a tire swing which can spin in a circle in either a clockwise or counter-clockwise direction. Any time your child moves his head upside-down or at an incline is vestibular movement. Input to the vestibular system can last in the body for up to four hours.

Why does my daughter hate to have her hair washed and her teeth brushed?

One of the most common questions I am asked is about hair, teeth, and grooming activities. We must complete these activities every day, and when there is trouble or anxiety surrounding them a stressful situation can result. I know and live with the fear of getting ready every day with my younger son. He is known to have a great deal of anxiety surrounding his hair and face. Each day I fear the time for grooming tasks. Just as with the seams and textures of clothing, our children may perceive input to the face, hair, and hands as physically painful. When something is painful, our bodies go into a "flight-or-fight" response. We may have sweating, increases in heart rate, and feelings of panic that may cause us great fear and avoidance of the situation. If the touch of the water on your child's hair or face is perceived as painful, burning, or sharp, then it causes a reaction similar to when your child feels pain. The same is true for brushing teeth. The water temperature, texture of the gritty toothpaste, or feeling of the brush along the inside of his mouth may each be overwhelming for him. The fear of the activity builds and then a tantrum can result.

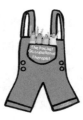 ## Out of the POCKET Activity

Since we must complete grooming activities on a daily basis to maintain hygiene, this area is critical to understand and for helping your child to become as comfortable as possible. The main technique is to allow your child to control as much as possible. Permit her to choose the toothbrush color or hardness of the bristles. Allow her to practice on her doll or favorite toy. Let her choose the flavor of the toothpaste. Make a schedule for her so that she can see a start time and end time for grooming. For example, give her three minutes to brush her teeth. Set a timer for her so that she can see that it will end.

See "Out of the POCKET Tips" for everyday activities in Chapter 6 for more suggestions regarding daily routines such as bathing, dressing, and hair washing.

Why does my child hate loud or unexpected noises?

On a daily basis, our auditory system is bombarded with a plethora of sounds. We must decide which is important to us at the time and which isn't. When a classroom is quiet, we can hear the sound of our teacher's footsteps, the child next to us tapping his fingers on the desk, someone sharpening her pencil, and so on. The auditory system can be protective to us. When we are sleeping, the one system that remains alert is the auditory system. This is because we need to determine if someone has broken a window, our baby is crying for food, or there is a fire alarm. We are awakened by certain sounds that we perceive and associate with danger to protect us from harm. Likewise, we screen sounds during the day. Sounds are directly connected with emotions. The sound of our mother's voice is recognized when we are infants and sounds we do not like can cause negative reactions. Think of nails running along a chalkboard. If you do not like this sound, you experience physical manifestations such as chills, goose pimples, and facial grimace (frowning or wrinkling of your face). This is a natural response to the sound. We have been given the auditory system to help us to survive in our world.

If a child is running on a heightened or hypo-sensitive sensory state, he may be extremely sensitive to many sounds and have difficulty blocking some of them out. When he is doing his homework, he may be distracted by sounds such as the lawnmower outside, children playing down the street, or even a siren passing by. He may be unable to concentrate due to every sound having the same intensity. Some children, like my older son, are extremely sensitive to unexpected sounds. Fire alarms, dogs barking, and thunder can be unpredictable and come at times when he least expects them. When an unexpected fire drill occurs at school, he has a great deal of anxiety and the feeling of panic. Remember that this can cause physical symptoms such as sweating, increased heart rate, and the fight-or-flight protective reactions. One time, we were in a hotel (oddly enough at a conference for children with autism) and the fire alarm went off at five a.m. He panicked and ran out of our hotel room heading for the emergency stairwell. This happened so quickly that we lost track of him in the confusion. He was five years old. The memory of the event caused him great anxiety and now, at 12 years of age, he refuses to stay at any hotel with a fire alarm that is similar to the one in the room that fateful day. It is so important to remember that our past experiences coupled with our current sensory alertness/state play a critical role in our function in daily life.

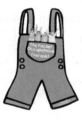

Out of the POCKET Activity

When a child is fearful of sounds, there are several things we can do to help. One of my favorite things is to allow the child to make a list of the sounds that frighten her. Do not make fun of or make light of any sound on the list. Remember, everyone is different! If possible, allow your child to control the sounds on the list, such as the hairdryer or vacuum cleaner. There is a CD called *Sound-Eaze* that is designed to give children control of sounds that they otherwise wouldn't be able to tolerate. It contains fireworks, thunder, dog barks, sirens, and fire drills among others. There is a *School-Eaze* version with school sounds included. Each sound is set to a rhythm and sometimes music. The music and then the rhythm each fade out, leaving only the sound. The child can then control the volume of the sound as she wishes. I created the CDs for my own children with the help of a music therapist, behavior therapist, and speech therapist. They can be purchased at www.route2greatness.com.

Other options for children with auditory (sound) sensitivity are to use noise-cancelling headphones. They block out outside noises thus allowing a quieter environment. Listening to calming music is helpful. Setting aside an area where it is quiet and with fewer distractions for tasks such as homework is a wonderful idea and adds the consistency of a routine and comfortable area to work in.

What is a sensory diet?

A sensory diet is a wonderful tool in helping to organize a child's sensory system. It is not a food diet, but rather an activity diet. The diet is specially tailored for every individual's sensory needs. The first step in making the diet is to ask the caregiver to keep a journal or list of the child's day. Note any "meltdowns" or tantrums; list times where any hyper-activity is noted; write about activities which cause joy and which cause frustration; ask the teacher to note behavior while seated at the desk or in circle time; note any difficulties with transitions; write about what kinds of movement your child prefers during non-structured time; note preferred and non-preferred foods; and jot down how bedtime and sleep routines look on a daily basis. I recommend keeping the journal for a week.

Meet with your OT and discuss the journal with her. She will then make a daily schedule of activities that should be completed at specific times during the day. There may be information about which kinds of foods to pack for snack and lunchtime. (We already know that chewing on crunchy and chewy snacks is generally calming and that drinking through a small straw is super for oral-input, calming, and giving proprioceptive input to the oral-motor musculature.) The diet is designed to maintain the sensory system's level of alertness at that "just right" state throughout the day so that sensory information is better processed and an appropriate output is formed. The sensory diet may be changed if an activity doesn't have the desired effect or doesn't seem to be working for your child. The beauty of the sensory diet is that it is specially designed for your child and it has an excellent success rate when followed as the OT prescribes it.

What is repetitive play?
What is self-regulation?

Children who have autism often find repeating the same behavior over and over to be soothing and calming.

My son used to flip over his baby walker and spin the wheels for hours. He reacted negatively when we took the toy away. Repetitive play provides children with a sense of predictability which seems to comfort them. We permitted my son to play with the toy, but limited the time he did so. Self-regulation is anything a child does to help stop impulsive behavior. So, when a child is "regulated" he is able to delay impulsive behavior and think about the next steps and results of his behavior. Regulation is the child's ability to calm himself down or initiate activities to make himself happy. It's quite a complex process. Social-emotional self-regulation involves following community rules and conforming to regulations individually and in a group setting. Cognitive self-regulation is the ability to learn and develop. To achieve self-regulation, a child must first be aware of his own emotions. He must then learn to manage them, or to learn that he is able to control those emotions. To have control, a child must think about how emotions may affect behavior and then consider safety. Think about a toddler who is two years old. His behavior is emotionally driven and he does not consider (or is not yet capable of thinking about) how lying on the toy store floor will affect his own safety. Behavior and desires to play with a certain toy take over his entire body and he immediately acts upon them.

Most children with autism have difficulty with planning, organizing, stopping impulses, and thinking ahead about consequences. In order to function in society, we need to consider how our behavior impacts others and further control our impulses and suppress them when necessary. Forming a replacement behavior or adapting to the environment is difficult for people who have autism.

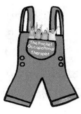

Out of the POCKET Activity

Children who have autism often lack awareness of their own body.

It's helpful to teach children where and when a particular behavior IS and IS NOT appropriate. Each behavior should be taught separately. As this takes time and many strategies, I recommend enlisting the help of a trained cognitive behavioral therapist or psychologist who is trained and experienced working with children who have autism.

Specific strategies need to be taught to children in order to help them to deal with emotions and impulses.

There is a neurological reason behind the difficulty children with autism experience. They are not trying to be difficult or acting badly in order to gain attention, their brains are lacking certain skill sets.

Why does my child refuse to touch certain items such as metal, coins, zippers, etc.?

My son avoids touching any metal at all costs. He has become an expert at using his feet to open door knobs and flush toilets. He does not like the feeling of metal nor can he tolerate the smell of metal. The use of coins also presents a great deal of difficulty for him. There are many strategies we use to assist him. He has learned to take deep breaths when he must touch metal. Afterwards, he visualizes a scent or smell he enjoys. When he is able, he quickly goes to the restroom to wash (scour) his hands.

Some children are not able to control their fear of metal. I suggest writing a social story about metal and that it cannot cause damage to our body. It's important to truly listen to your child as his fears are real to him. Do not dismiss any concern just because you do not experience the same feelings. Use gloves if your child cannot tolerate metal or until therapy is started. An alternative is to carry a baby wipe in your pocket and wipe off your child's hand until it can be washed with soap and water.

Why does my child follow straight lines with his eyes?

When my son was five he began to tilt his head, squint his eyes, and lean in toward any wall, table, or object that had a straight line. He followed the line with his head cocked sideways and didn't seem aware of his other surroundings. This behavior was repeated until I distracted him or told him to stop.

I've seen hundreds of clients who have autism and who repeat this same behavior. The first thing I recommend is to see a developmental optician. They are specifically trained in not only the vision but also the function of the eyes as they work individually and together. Additionally, your child may be craving sensory input to his face or oral-motor muscles.

Never force a child to make eye contact. Many people who have autism and are able to communicate report that it is too difficult to look into someone's eyes. Making eye contact is quite overwhelming so may cause over-stimulation since they may be hyper aware of many other things in the environment. When a child is avoiding looking at your eyes it does not mean he is not listening to you. Simply ask for a verbal confirmation that your child is listening.

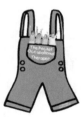

Out of the POCKET Activities

Remember that when your child is attempting to self-regulate in any way, his body is "telling you" that it's out of sensory sync and needs help. Learning to read your child's body language is critical to detecting dysregulation.

- Provide a regular activity schedule of deep pressure, wearing weighted or compression clothing; use Lycra fabric to wrap your child up like a hot dog in a bun.

- Complete activities in a mirror such as putting a dab of chocolate, pudding, or whipping cream on his face and using the tongue to lick it off.

- Drink liquids from a coffee stirrer or tiny straw. These activities encourage "heavy work" of the muscles of the mouth and cheeks.

- Complete a nice relaxing massage to face and cheeks. Include listening to classical music or rhythmic movement while placing a weighted bag full of rice over his eyes for relaxation.

My child flaps her hands and makes movements with her arms. Why?

People who have autism often have difficulty regulating their sensory system (see the "What is Self-Regulation" section). Movement of hands in flapping, wiggling, and other ways helps a person who has autism to calm themselves. There are times that children need more movement to organize the nervous system or the brain. It's perfectly fine that a child is attempting to soothe herself. Education of others around your child is important so that they have a better understanding of "why" your child is moving.

- Work with your child to do "heavy work" activities such as pulling, pushing, lifting, and carrying. Complete an obstacle course while crawling.

- Do Yoga activities which require putting weight on the arms such as downward dog.

- Play with dough and form letters, numbers, shapes, foods, etc.

- Encourage your child to complete self-stimulatory behavior in private if possible. For example, my teenage son prefers to move his hands in his room, in the restroom at school, or in the car when he becomes overwhelmed. In fact, we created a card he may give the teacher when he needs to leave the classroom. It's in the "accommodations" section of his IEP and it's been an excellent tool for him.

Why does my child line up his toys or sort toys instead of playing with them?

This is one of the most common questions I'm asked on a daily basis. Remember that a "hallmark" sign of autism is routine/insisting on completing the same activities on a repetitive basis. Playing in a repetitive manner can be organizing to a child. Lining up toys is a predictable and soothing activity. It's always the same and can be repeated over and over. It's important for us to allow our children to line toys up BUT limiting the time spent doing so. I suggest use of a visual timer to provide a beginning and end point to the behavior. Additionally, sit down with your child and play with the objects in a different way. Encourage the toys to slide down a make-believe ramp or get "dirty" in some muddy water. Ask kids to help "clean" up the toys with a toothbrush and bucket of water. This type of play encourages imagination and also helps with sensory processing and motor skills. Remember that adding regular sensory activities such as pushing, pulling, lifting and carrying are important to help a child's body to feel more regulated.

My child repeats the same phrase over and over or my child repeats what others or television programs say

Repetition is comforting for everyone. Repeating the same words or phrases is called echolalia. Young babies often imitate others in order to learn language. This may be one reason children with autism complete this behavior. Another reason is that this is another example of a self-stimulatory behavior. It's similar to the lining up of toys, but has an auditory component or one that your child can hear.

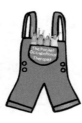

Out of the POCKET Activities

- Repeat the same phrase with your child and then expand on the words. For example, if your child says, "The train went, 'Choo Choo' as it chugged down the track," you might say, "The train went 'beep beep' as it chugged down the road in a hurry." Playing a game with language is a fun way to help your child.

- Clap out the words or use movement. It's a fun way to increase interaction and add a kinetic (movement) component.

- Give your child a cheek massage, chew a hard snack, or try any other sensory activity for oral-motor input as listed in Chapter 3 on Feeding Difficulty.

- Adding music, singing, or rhymes is a fun way to play with words.

Remember to get down to your child's physical height level and play alongside of her to begin. Getting too close may give your child anxiety, so sit next to her and imitate what she's doing and gradually add the techniques listed above. Go slow and have fun!

Why does my child dislike wind, rain, and getting wet?

The child's tactile system is in charge of receiving and perceiving touch on the skin. If a child is hypersensitive to light touch, he may fear water. Instead of thinking, "My body is wet right now, but it will dry soon or I will use a towel to dry off," our children may feel pain or fear and experience a threat/danger response of fight-or-flight. Once that occurs, children may experience a panic response. For example, my son actually refuses to leave our home if there are clouds or a threat of rain in the sky. He has not yet learned how to cope with the anxiety he feels when it's raining. Remember that raindrops give a light touch and are unpredictable. Sometimes the rain pours straight down and other times it's blowing toward the side. An umbrella does not provide full coverage.

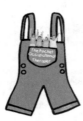

Out of the POCKET Activities

- Acknowledge the child's fear and provide understanding.

- Use swim goggles so that rain or water does not go into the eyes.

- Complete some heavy work activities before bathing or showering. In our home, our children take off dirty clothes and place them into a laundry basket. I added bean bags to the basket so that the kids' muscles must work harder as they carry the items to the laundry area.

- Allow children to wear a swim suit in the shower/tub.

- Add relaxing scents to the water such as vanilla or lavender.

- Give your child a watering can so that she may wash her toys.

- Purchase a raincoat and call it a cool name such as "The Super Rain Shield."

- Allow your child to wear a hat or cover his head.

- Always ensure he has an umbrella in his backpack to help avoid a sensory-related meltdown if it rains while walking to bus or home.

My child is in constant motion. Why is my child fidgeting his hands/feet?

Your child may move his hands and feet constantly: fidget; spin, jump or twirl; or run around in circles without getting dizzy. A child who has hypo (low) sensory response often requires more of a stimulus or activity in order to register it in his sensory system. Remember that rhythmic or repetitive movement can be quite calming. Also, hanging upside down provides input to the spine, muscles, and vestibular system. A child may need more of this type of input to regulate or maintain a calm and orderly state. There is a category of sensory processing disorder called "sensory craving." A child who craves is in a constant need of activity which will provide touch, position, or movement to her body. Sometimes, a child who is a craver appears to have attention disorders.

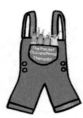

Out of the POCKET Activities

- Provide regular sensory activities (a sensory diet).

- Include items such as large therapy/Yoga balls, swinging in a linear (side to side or back and forth) movement, trampolines, and obstacle course items in daily play.

- Use fidget toys such as the Tangle®, Koosh balls, therapy putty or dough.

- Have your child wear compression garments such as SPIO.

- Add chores which include pulling, pushing, lifting, and carrying. Set the dinner table, move chairs, vacuum, carry laundry or sweep with a broom.

- Consider purchase of a BOSU® ball for balance activities which force the body to work harder to maintain an upright position.

- Use vibrating pillows or weighted items such as blankets, vests, hats or lap pads.

- Jump rope or play hopscotch.

- It's OK for kids to invert their heads against gravity. Movement upside down is powerful to the child's sensory system. SAFETY FIRST, though…all movement against gravity should be child-directed. The child's sensory system may benefit from this motion for up to 6–8 hours!

Why does my child get upset in the grocery store and refuse to go to restaurants?

Our family is quite familiar with both situations. We have experienced many sensory-related tantrums in stores. Most stores have fluorescent lighting which can affect us in negative ways. This type of lighting flickers and can make noise which many children who are hypersensitive to sound are able to hear. Additionally, the store is a very unpredictable setting. People are moving in all directions, music is playing, sounds are random and can be loud. The temperatures in grocery stores can vary from section to section which may adversely affect a child who is sensitive to temperature.

Restaurants are also unpredictable and are full of scents, noises, flavors, and visual stimuli. Additionally, patrons move about randomly.

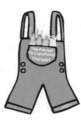 ## Out of the POCKET Activities

- Noise-cancelling headphones are excellent for stores, restaurants, sporting events, airplane trips and many more settings.

- Bring along a comfort item such as a stuffed toy. Our son prefers dice and brings one for each hand to help him with transitions.

- Allow your child to push the shopping cart for heavy work/calming activity.

- Give your child a mini shopping list or ask her to reach for and give you the items on your list.

- Allow your child to wear a jacket or long-sleeved shirt for those stores which have coolers and frozen sections.

- Have your child wear compression garments under clothing such as those made by SPIO®.

- Set up a backseat "sensory area." Place a weighted lap pad or vibratory pillow, a fidget toy, or a "find-it" type visual activity. (The toy is usually a cylinder filled with colored plastic pieces. There are child-friendly items floating in the plastic and your child needs to shake and turn the toy in order to find each item.) Play relaxing classical music or those CDs with heavy and low drum beats. Sacred-Earth Drums is a great example.

- Allow your child to play a game at the restaurant table. We play I spy, tic-tac-toe, or the what's missing game. Place five items on the table (such as the salt and pepper shaker, a sugar packet, ketchup, and a straw). Give your child 30 seconds to look at the items. Remove one while he covers his eyes and ask which item is missing. Distraction is always a great tool!

• Ask for a coffee stirrer and allow your child to drink from the stirrer. This is a great way to incorporate "heavy work" to the mouth.

Why is my child walking on her toes?

Children often walk on their toes. However, when toe-walking leads to tight heel cords (Achilles tendons), therapy may be in order. When he was six, my son required casts on both of his feet. He had walked on his toes for many years and we weren't sure what to do. The casts were changed by a physical therapist weekly and provided a gentle stretch to his heel cords. There are many ways to help your child to learn to use his entire foot when walking.

If your child has sensory processing disorder, he may be avoiding making full foot contact on the floor due to a sensitivity to touch on his skin. Our hands and feet are designed to be extra sensitive in order to protect us from becoming injured and subsequently getting an infection. Some of our children are hyper (over) responsive to tactile input. As a result, they avoid bearing weight on their foot and use as little surface area as possible. As we walk in bare feet, we feel many textures: wood, carpet, laminate, concrete, sand, dirt, grass, wet areas, step on toys, etc.

Talk to your child to determine the root cause of toe-walking. Remember that walking on the toes for a prolonged period of time causes the heel cords to become tightened.

Encourage children to wear socks and/or shoes indoors to avoid tactile input.

Use massagers or hands to provide a deep pressure massage to your child's feet.

Stretch his feet gently every evening. Here's how: ask your child to lie on the bed with his toes up. Sit facing your child's feet. Place one hand on the back of the lower leg and over the muscle. Press the other hand on the bottom of your child's foot and gently push it toward the ceiling. Hold for a count of three and release. It's important to provide a slow and gentle stretch and to avoid causing pain. The idea is to give a slight stretch to the heels every day to gradually increase and/or maintain flexibility of the feet.

Play games while walking on heels only. We do this in the clinic as we play hide and seek, do a fun obstacle course, or make silly animal sounds.

If your child refuses to walk bare-footed, slowly encourage sensory play in different bins filled with texture. Ask your child to sit on a chair while he places his feet into a sand bin to find toys with his toes or use smooth rocks and pretend fish to explore with his feet.

Chapter 6

Behavior and Transitions During Daily Activities

What is behavior?

Often, we think of behavior as a tantrum or action our child does to get attention. However, behavior by definition in the Merriam-Webster Dictionary is: "a: the manner of conducting oneself; b: anything that an organism does involving action and response to stimulation; c: the response." Children respond to their environment. From birth, we are bombarded with lights, sounds, textures, and touches. It is our response to these things (stimuli) that helps us to survive in the world. For instance, when a baby cries for his bottle, his caregiver feeds him. He learns that his actions have consequences and then either repeats them or tries something else. You may have learned that there is a texture or sound, such as nails scraping on a chalkboard, that bothers you and thus you avoid it. Children who have learning disabilities or difficulty navigating the world around them may have difficulty responding appropriately to things around them. In addition, if the child feels threatened in any way, he may very well respond to protect himself.

My son has impulsive reactions to loud noises. When he hears a loud unexpected noise, he runs around and screams loudly. He does not consider those around him, nor his own safety. We call a response to "protect" our body a fight-or-flight response. Fight-or-flight responses are our body's innate or in-born responses to something we perceive as a threat or danger to us. It is through these responses that we are able to protect ourselves from something dangerous or thought to be dangerous or threatening. So, my son's behavior is in response to an outside stimulus, and whether it is socially acceptable behavior or not is meaningless to him; he copes in the best way he knows how and that is to flee the situation and scream loudly while doing so.

It is my belief that a child can succeed when given the opportunity, and when she has a response to something (behavior), there is usually a reason. As clinicians and caregivers it is our job to find that reason. Infants cry because they are unable to talk. In the same way, our children's actions reflect something that they may not be able to accurately describe to us. This concept is especially important when dealing with a child with a special need or with decreased verbal skills. These children simply do not have the words to let us know what they are experiencing. We are left to be detectives and find out what the root of a behavior may be. It is always good to have a team approach and good communication with therapists, teachers, and so on, so that we can acquire the "big picture" of our child's issues. Note: I am not referring to a child in this chapter who is acting out solely for attention or to purposefully defy an adult or authority. What I am addressing is a child with a sensory processing dysfunction or other special need which interferes with the ability to appropriately react and interact with our environment and surroundings.

A child may not want to go to gym class because the coach uses a whistle or the room has an echo. The child may act out before gym class due to anxiety about the upcoming event. He may not be able to verbalize this fear, but will throw a tantrum in math class for no apparent reason. If we are to fully understand him and provide him with the skills to succeed, we must take the time to understand the situation.

Another child may refuse to participate in circle time. She may throw herself onto the floor and kick when the announcement is made to join her peers on the carpet. Other children may stare or comment, and the teacher or aide may solely look at her behavior at that time instead of attempting to determine why she may indeed be acting out. She may not like the way the carpet feels on her body or the closeness she feels to the other children in the circle. It may be the lighting in that area of the classroom, or there may have been a fire drill at the last circle time. If her verbal skills are decreased, we may have to spend extra time with simple yes/no questions in order to get to the bottom of the issue.

Why is giving a child choices SO important?

I make many choices every day. I do not like it when someone forces me to do something that I do not want to do. Our children are the same way. They like the freedom to make choices. In fact, society has labeled "the terrible twos" as a time when children are notorious for acting upon the choices that they themselves have made. By making choices that cause success, confidence is built to explore. The desire to repeat a positive interaction with the environment grows stronger. When we make a choice, we react to something in our environment. This is our way of interacting with the world around us. So, how do we get our children to do something that is "non-preferred" or that they don't want to do? We offer them choices. For instance, you may have carrots or peas tonight; you may take a bath or shower. Either way, the desired outcome is met but your child feels the power of choosing his interaction with the world, although children on the autism spectrum or with sensory processing disorder may become overwhelmed if too many choices are given. In addition, a choice given along with a visual cue is important.

The caveat is that a negative behavior that is reinforced may cause repeated negative behaviors. A child who sneaks out of his bedroom window and is not caught will likely repeat the behavior simply because nothing negative resulted. If you read this book and learn one thing, I'd like it to be that autism or having a special need is no excuse for bad behavior. There needs to be a consequence for negative behavior if you expect your child to live successfully in society.

Why does changing our routine make my child so upset?

Yesterday, I was driving with my son. I quickly decided to make a right turn to run a quick errand. I had not provided warning of the change. He proceeded to have an hour long tantrum in which he hit himself, screamed obscenities, and tried to escape the vehicle. We all lead busy lives and make long- and short-term decisions. Every day, we need to be flexible and realize that sometimes adaptability is necessary to function. Additionally, as we interact with others, they make quick decisions too and we must adapt in social situations. Unfortunately, difficulty remaining flexible is one of the traits of autism. We all crave routine and predictability, yet understand that split-second decisions are necessary.

SAFETY FIRST: always anticipate difficult behavior and have a safety plan in place. Stress hormones are released when humans become upset and cause us to seek out safety without considering consequences. In the vehicle we enable the child escape safety locks. At home, we have high locks on our doors and use devices to limit the distance in which our windows open. The desire to escape the situation comes fast and furiously. We must protect our children.

Try to give as much notice as possible.

Repeat words such as, "I know that you are upset and angry that we made this turn. I understand and let's take a few deep breaths together." Providing validation to our children's feelings is important.

Distract with a sensory activity bag. We keep the bags in our purse, car, family's homes, etc. In the bag is a form of vibratory input such as massagers or Z-Vibes. A sensory bag with putty and small toys buried in the putty, a visual/emotional chart, and fidget toy are also contained in the bag.

Life will force us to make quick decisions, so make a plan together with your child about what to do when he's upset. Include calm-down techniques and an emotion/feeling chart, and practice how to take deep cleansing breaths.

Why does my daughter hold it together at school all day but have a meltdown as soon as she gets home?

I encourage you to be conscious of your feelings and emotions during a workday or social outing. We change our body to fit the situation and this requires a great deal of energy. Schools are full of colors, noises, learning, social interactions and more. Often children with autism "hold it together" at school and function at their best. The requirement of energy and awareness is great. As soon as children get into a comfortable setting and are with someone who loves and accepts them for who they truly are, they are able to release the stress they've been holding in all day.

Provide a break for your child as soon as he gets home. Choose an area in which to place weighted blankets, calm music or fidget toys, or create movement opportunities such as jumping on a trampoline, running outside, or completing fun activities such as a crawling obstacle course. Remember to use as many muscles as possible to release extra energy. Allow the break right after school and before homework time is attempted. Our entire family engages in a fun and relaxing activity when we arrive home from work and school. Activities include a family game of tag, swimming, playing basketball, pretending to drum to different beats, listening to rhythmic music and imitating each other's dance moves. Everyone needs a sensory break after a long day.

What is a transition?

Transitions happen thousands of times each day. You move from your bed to the bathroom, from brushing your teeth to combing your hair. So, a transition is simply a change from one activity to another. Most times, a smooth transition happens when you move to an activity that you prefer and a bumpy transition may result to an activity that is non-preferred. Unfortunately, children with autism may have great difficulty with transitions. We find that children with autism have difficulty with abstract concepts such as time. If a child doesn't understand what is coming next, she may have increased anxiety which may cause a negative behavior. The magnitude of the anxiety increases when a child cannot express verbally the fear of the unknown or anxiety about an upcoming activity. It is due to this that we must implement a visual chart and relaxation techniques along with practice.

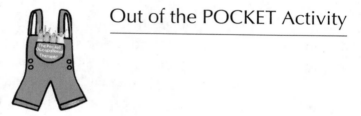

Out of the POCKET Activity

Making a chart of activities with visuals is important to helping with transitions. The cheapest way is to take pictures with your own camera and place them in order of time. If you desire, a lamination machine is helpful and can be purchased at any local office supply store. Remember to purchase extra laminating sheets for the future. Velcro tabs can be placed on the back of the pictures so that you may rearrange the pictures depending on the events. For an evening routine: take a picture of your child's pajamas, a picture of his toothbrush and toothpaste, one of the toilet, and one of his bed. Place them in order and review them with him before he begins. Use words such as "first, next, after that, and at the end." Most children enjoy handing you the picture after the activity is finished to obtain a simple reward such as a smile or a high five. Some children put the pictures onto the schedule as they are completed to see their progress. Either way may work with your child. In fact, one of my children prefers to take off the pictures and the other prefers to place the pictures onto the chart as he's finished.

Sometimes an activity needs to be broken down into specific steps for your child. So, for hand washing, take a picture of the faucet, then one of your child turning on the water, one of her using soap, another of her turning off the faucet, and finally one of her drying her hands. You can laminate the pictures and place them onto a chart near the sink. It is extremely rewarding for both you and your child to watch skills develop and independence blossom.

Encouraging positive behavior during everyday activities

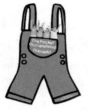

Out of the POCKET Tips

Dressing

- Give choices about color of shirt and pants (remember that you are in control of the color and limit choices to two or three that actually match).

- Use a visual schedule for dressing and undressing. This should be step by step with as many pictures of the clothing as possible.

- Give your child a choice of which article of clothing goes on first.

- Allow your child to choose specific types of clothing. DO NOT force your child to wear tags or clothing with wording on them if he does not like them. You will have a struggle of power from the start due to his limited ability to tolerate the clothing. Slowly work into the clothing using techniques outlined in Chapter 5 or with your occupational therapist.

I purchased a five-drawer plastic unit from my local home improvement store. I labeled it from the top drawer to the bottom drawer to help him to understand what article of clothing he needed to put on in which order. The top drawer has a bright number one sticker on it. This drawer holds underwear; drawer number two contains his shirts (I re-stock the clothing bins based on the seasons); drawer number three contains pants or shorts; drawer number four has socks; and drawer five holds shoes. He is able to get dressed in order with concrete visuals with both the numbers on the drawers and the location of them—starting at the top and working to the bottom. There are two choices in each drawer and I pre-stock them so that either choice will match.

Bathing

- Allow your child to choose a bath or shower.

- Play soft or relaxing music during bathing.

- Allow a transition item or toy into the tub that makes her feel comfortable.

- Use colored bath tablets to turn water a color your child chooses.

- Use a colored bath towel that she has chosen.

- Use a drop-in capsule containing a sponge toy that expands in water. These are sold in packages containing various colors and shapes. Allow her to choose a capsule each bath time.

Hair washing

One of the most frequent questions I receive is regarding hair washing and cutting. Try the techniques below and repeat them. Be consistent and try not to become frustrated with your child. He is trying his best too!

- Use a hand-held shower to allow your child to control the water's direction.

- Give him a cup and allow him to rinse his hair.

- Give his scalp a gentle massage before trying to wash his hair as a warm-up.

- Allow him to wash your hair or his favorite toy's hair.

- My son prefers me to give him a countdown of how many rinses I am going to do. I usually begin with ten and let him use his fingers to count down the rinses.

- Allow him to hold a dry washcloth over his face. This may give him a feeling of control.

- Use gentle relaxing music or sing a repetitive song. Encourage him to sing along.

- Use a visual schedule: first we pour water over your hair; next we use shampoo to rub your hair; at the end we rinse your hair and we are all done.

Haircuts

Typically children experience anxiety surrounding haircuts. The feeling of being helpless in a chair while a stranger is working on your hair is an unfamiliar situation for children. They do not have control over what the stylist is doing and anxiety results. Preparation and relaxation are key to success.

- Make sure to brush or comb your child's hair regularly at home. Encourage her to help you.

- I prefer to meet with the stylist before I bring my son in. I give a mini-interview to determine if she's empathetic or has experience with children who do not like having their hair cut.

- Take your child for a visit to the salon at a time other than during a haircut.

- Going to a salon specializing in children's haircuts is a good idea. Try to go first thing in the morning when it's not as busy and stimulating. They often cost more, but the individual attention is well worth it. Our local child's salon allows my son to choose a video and then watch it with or without headphones during the haircut.

- Allow your child to suck on a lollipop or chew crunchy snacks or gum during the haircut.

- Provide gentle scalp massage before the haircut to prepare her.

- Provide a visual schedule of the haircut: first your hair will be sprayed with a water bottle; then the stylist will use scissors to trim your hair; next she will brush your hair, etc.

- If your child does not like a hairdryer, let your stylist know prior to the appointment.

- Allow your child to choose which cape she will wear—if she will wear one at all.

- Give a reward that your child has chosen after the haircut.

- Cut your child's hair at home or ask local stylists if they are willing to come to your home.

- Have another peer go with you and your child and get haircuts together. Go out for a fun activity afterward.

Nail clipping

- Try clipping the nails when he's asleep.

- Apply gentle pressure to the nail beds (cuticle area) before and during clipping.

- Sing a rhythmic song that your child can sing along to.

- Use a nail file instead of clippers. Sometimes the sound of either the clippers or the file may cause a great deal of anxiety so make sure to ask your child which he prefers. Ask him at a time other than during the activity to give him a chance to provide an answer while not having anxiety in the moment.

- Have a countdown of nails and blast-off at the end with a fun activity!

- Try cutting nails after a bath. The nails actually soften and are easier to cut.

Teeth brushing

- Allow your child to choose her toothbrush color.

- Give a vibrating or electric toothbrush.

- Try a toothbrush that plays a song while brushing. This song can be sung prior to the actual brushing so that she will know what is coming up.

- Allow her to brush her favorite doll's teeth.

- Offer flavored toothpaste.

- Set a visual timer to let her know how long she has left for the activity.

Doctor or dentist visits

- Interview your doctor or dentist without your child to determine if there's a good personality match. You want a physician who will listen to your questions and schedule extra time if necessary.

- Take your child to the office for a visit to look around and familiarize himself with the office.

- Make a list of questions that you want to ask ahead of time. Ask a friend to come and watch your child after the examination is over to ensure you have adequate time to have questions answered.

- Make a visual schedule and review it with your child before the visit. First we will enter the waiting room, next we will hear our name called, then we will be weighed and measured, and so on. Take actual pictures if possible of the equipment and laminate them onto a schedule. Place Velcro on the back of each picture. Have your child either tear off the pictures as the activity is completed or put the pictures onto the schedule as they are completed to see her progress. Either way may work with your child. In fact, one of my children prefers to take off the pictures and the other prefers to place the pictures onto the chart as he's finished. You'll need to practice this at home prior to the visit.

- Write a letter to the doctor, stylist, or dentist prior to your visit. I have written many letters for my clients regarding sensory processing difficulties and communication issues. It is perfectly acceptable to ask your pediatrician or therapist to compose a letter regarding any medical diagnosis your child may have. There are times when a letter is necessary in order for you not to speak about your child's difficulties in front of him. Also, caregivers who do not feel comfortable verbally discussing their child's difficulties may find handing out a letter to be less stressful. Letters may be written to address specific issues, such as transition difficulties and resulting anxiety, possible aggression issues, and decreased verbal skills. It is often helpful to include a resource such as a website so that the recipient may look up specific information in order to better understand the situation.

Here is an example letter:

Dear _____,

My child has been diagnosed with an autism spectrum disorder. Sometimes he has difficulty with new situations and strangers. If you notice that he is uncomfortable, please work with him and help him to try to understand his environment. This may mean giving him very specific instructions and even giving him a picture or chart of what is coming up next. He may need some extra time to adjust and become familiar with his environment so please be patient with him. I am excited to work with you!

Please visit www._____ for more information.

Thank you!

_____

Making your expectations clear

Autism or any special need is no excuse for bad behavior. A child who spits at her therapist solely in defiance needs to have a distinct consequence. Make your expectations clear and place a written or picture list of behaviors which are not acceptable. The sign should be clearly posted where your child can see it and you should review it with her regularly. If a rule is broken, the consequences need to be consistent as empty threats will not work with any child. Following through is the key to getting results.

Rewards are important to all of us. You work for a paycheck, your dog sits to get a treat, and so on. Children are no exception. A special food, stickers, praise, trips to the park, or extra play time after therapy, are excellent rewards. Discuss your expectations with your child and when she follows through with good behavior, be sure to reward her. In my clinic, I have posted a list of rules. The rules are posted with pictures:

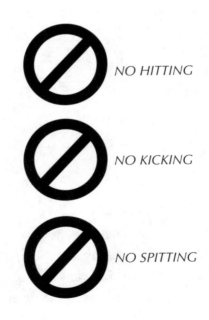

NO HITTING

NO KICKING

NO SPITTING

Transition tools and resources—final thoughts

There are many wonderful tools to assist children with transitions. One of my favorites is a visual timer. There are several different types, but all provide a visual representation of the amount of time left before an activity is over. Remember that time is an abstract concept and, for our children, time is difficult to grasp and fully understand. You can make a chart that looks like a stop light with a red, yellow, and green circle. When there is a certain amount of time left, then keep the green circle on the chart. As time is winding down, take green off and place the yellow circle on. When time is finished, take yellow off and place red on. It is imperative that you allow your child enough time to complete an activity. No one likes to be rushed and children who already may be having a difficult time with transitioning need extra patience.

A transition object can be very helpful. Your child can carry a familiar object or toy with him when moving from activity to activity. This may give him a sense of comfort and stability in the changing situation. Allow him to choose the object.

Make all directions clear and concise. Many children have difficulty processing commands, especially when they are verbal commands. If the direction has too many words and not enough concrete examples, a child may not understand exactly what you meant. Speak as few words as possible and, whenever you can, use gestures. The visual charts described in the "What is a transition?" section should be used whenever possible.

Chapter 7

Toilet Training

How do I know when my child is ready to begin toileting?

Toileting progresses from a reflexive act to a cognitive act as babies grow and develop. Typically developing children show readiness to toilet train between the ages of 24–36 months. However, when parenting a child with special needs, professionals consider the developmental (or functional) age of the child versus the chronological age. Every child who begins toilet training must show signs of readiness. Therapists who work with children with special needs often create charts called elimination records to determine how long a child stays dry, times a child usually has bowel movements, and if a child is aware that he's soiled his diaper.

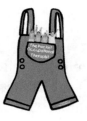

Out of the POCKET Tips

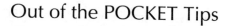

To be ready for toileting a child should:

- Demonstrate willingness to sit on the toilet with clothing on.

- Show ability to pull pants down independently.

- Be willing to wash her hands as this is critical for hygiene.

- Agree to wear regular underwear rather than diapers/pull-ups.

- Notice and/or look uncomfortable when he soils his diaper.

- Follow simple commands.

- Remain dry in diaper for up to two hours, including naps.

- Not be fearful of the bathroom or toilet.

Why does my son refuse to use the potty?

Our brains are hard-wired to protect our body from danger. Often, our current functional level is directly tied to the experiences we've had. Children who have sensory difficulty may be over- or under- responsive and, as a result, make a strong attempt to protect themselves from what is perceived as a dangerous situation. Additionally, children who have autism may exhibit social deficits or lack of empathy or even awareness of others' feelings. Socially, being a "big boy" may not be enough to motivate him as he may not have the desire to please others. Think of the many steps in toileting. For a child who has difficulty following commands, completing a process with so many steps can be simply overwhelming. Children with special needs may crave routines and schedules. Changing from having a bowel movement in a diaper or pull-up to going on the potty may appear daunting or bring resistance from the child. He may be labeled as controlling since he often feels so out of control. Using the toilet requires us to release the fecal matter and urine that our body does not need. However, the feeling we experience may cause a "loss" to the child. Also, the child may have experienced a situation that was perceived as scary or loud when using a toilet in the past. One of my clients, like many children I work with, was five when she began to use the toilet for bowel movements. She preferred the feeling of going into a pull-up as a way of feeling in control of her own body. This is extremely common for children who have sensory issues. She showed an intense fear of "a part of her" going into the toilet and being flushed away. Her parents used calming strategies to help her to breathe deeply and relax. Also, she used a small portable toilet and her parents slowly moved it from her bedroom to the bathroom.

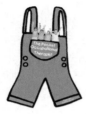

Out of the POCKET Tips

- Use a visual schedule for toileting.

- Read books designed for children who are toilet training. Examples available from Amazon® include:

    » *Let's Get This Potty Started*, by Dr Heather Wittenberg

    » *Going To The Potty*, by Mr. Rogers

    » *Your New Potty*, by Joanna Cole and Margaret Miller

    » *Everyone Poops*, by Taro Gomi

    » *Where's the Poop*, by Susan Hartung

    » *My Potty Reward Stickers*, by Tracy Foote

- Potty apps are now available for smart phones. Examples are Once Upon a Potty or Sym Trend ADL.

- Have a special potty toy and only allow your child to play with it when she's on the toilet. If she spends more than 20 minutes playing and not "going," put the toy aside and try again later.

- Some kids feel more in control when they sit backwards on the toilet. We even let our sons use a dry-erase marker to draw on the toilet!

- Allow kids to be naked while in the bathroom and during toileting attempts. Often children are concerned with getting messy or soiled.

- Use candles, scented oils, or non-chemical scents in order to set a relaxing environment.

- Express understanding and empathy instead of anger and frustration...remember that your child is fully aware of the situation.

- Use a sensory activity diet regularly to help the entire body.

- Ask your child if the temperature of the toilet seat or room is comfortable.

- Go to the same toilet when possible. Remember that routine is comforting to your child.

- Avoid public restrooms which can have loud hand dryers, unpredictable noises, and smells.

- Purchase a special bag of gifts for a child who is beginning toileting. Items to include may be: special wipes, toileting books, reward stickers, and a chart.

What are some toileting adaptations to try at home with my child?

Providing a safe and comfortable environment is critical to a child's willingness to use the toilet. For example, using the powder room versus the full bathroom will decrease distractions and provide a more cozy space for kids.

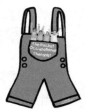

Out of the POCKET Tips

- Sit with clothes on to develop a comfort with the bathroom.

- Model toileting for your child if you feel comfortable doing so. Bring your child into the restroom with you to demonstrate the process and washing hands afterward.

- Try a soft toilet seat to improve comfort and alleviate the cold feeling that sitting on a standard toilet seat gives.

- Use a visual timer or toileting chart so children can see when the task ends. Examples of schedules may be found at:

  » www.freeprintablebehaviorcharts.htm

  » www.pottytrainingconcepts.com

  » www.autismspeaks.org

- Move all toileting supplies to the area where toilet training will occur. Providing consistency will assist children who have difficulty beginning a new skill.

- Use a physical support for children who feel as though they will "fall in." Grab bars or even use of a stool for propping feet up helps a child to feel secure.

- If flushing is an issue for your child, tape a cover onto the handle.

- Allow children to flush when they are ready. Use ready, set, GO! or any phrase the child creates.

- Tape a line on the wall as a visual for limiting toilet paper. Make a rule that only five sheets/squares of paper may be used at one time.

- Use a piece of cereal as a target for kids to aim at in the bowl.

- Try using food coloring in the water for a visual target and fun.

- Alter diapers by making a cut in the bottom. Begin with a hole then cut the diaper ¼ open, then ½ and so on.

Why is my child having bowel and bladder accidents often?

Our body is designed to function on its own. For example, we feel hunger and thirst automatically and we don't purposefully control our heart and kidneys. But we are aware of pain in the organs, such as when our heart flutters, or if we need to use the toilet. The internal organs are designed to function on their own. The "way we feel in the inside" is called *interoception*. Often children who are hypo (low) sensory responsive require more input in order for them to notice it. For example, a child didn't realize that he needed to urinate and wet his pants. So, children may not even recognize the need to eat, drink, urinate, etc.

Accidents will occur and it's important to remain calm and patient. *Praise, praise, praise* for positive attempts to use the toilet.

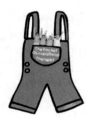

Out of the POCKET Tips

- Be patient and understanding toward your child. Do not yell or punish her if she has frequent accidents. Remember that every person wants to succeed and there may be a reason.

- Ask the pediatrician about possible medical explanations.

- Provide a consistent sensory-diet.

- Use a schedule to encourage regular trips to the toilet.

- Set a timer so that it alarms every two to three hours and the child gets used to stopping a preferred activity to use the toilet.

- Have your child use the toilet within 20 to 30 minutes after eating a meal and after drinking liquids.

- Read books about toilet training together and remember that every child develops on her own.

- Remember that constipation should be considered if your child does not have a bowel movement after two days. Consult your physician.

Chapter 8

Social Skills and Relationships

Why does my child refuse to go on play dates or spend time at the playground?

There may be many reasons why children with autism and/or sensory processing disorder, among others prefer to be alone or have one-on-one interactions. Many neurotypical people have difficulty or stress in social situations. When people gather together, they talk and laugh, hug or bump each other on purpose or accidentally and communicate. Remember that children with autism and SPD often have communication difficulty and trouble interpreting body language and social cues. Additionally, any unexpected bump or touch may feel painful or cause stress. Loud noises or the jumbled sounds of a group of people talking may be overwhelming.

Sensory processing disorder often causes children to experience fear when their body is moving against gravity. They do not like to be off of the ground in any way. The playground has high platforms that sometimes move and requires a certain level of "maturity" in processing activities and working against gravity's pull. Movement in any way when the head is upside-down or the body is off of the ground, such as riding a bicycle, is difficult for the child and is avoided.

Why does my child avoid affection from me or others?

Since I'm the mother to two children who have autism, I'm quite familiar with this question. I experience the same resistance from my boys and often become frustrated or feel sad since my sons are not affectionate and resist kisses and hugs. Through the years, I've met thousands of parents who feel the same way. There are alternative ways to show affection such as through sweet notes, drawing pictures, and making a "secret" code for love. My younger son does not enjoy hugs or touch of any type. We enjoy sitting next to each other to play Minecraft ® or one of his preferred games. It's a rare thing to see his eyes meet mine, but when they do it's the best feeling! He is a fan of Howie Mandel and as a result, we frequently bump fists. It's not a hug, but it's my son's way of telling me he loves me and enjoys our time together.

Many children who have autism experience hypersensitivity to light touch or any unexpected touch from others. This includes kisses, hugs, pats on the back. Other children may prefer to get a big squeeze for a hug vs. a light embrace. Discuss this with your therapist and your child. Learn the reasons why if possible. Most often, the child needs to begin a sensory activity diet (Chapter 5). Deep pressure is often calming and it's best to practice hugging before any family gathering or times when hugging relatives may be expected. Some ideas for children who need squeezes vs light touch are: SPIO® compression garments, hug vests, or weighted clothing. Additionally, light kisses on the cheek may throw your child into a sensory overload. Again, the light touch of a gentle kiss may be too stimulating for the child's sensory system. It's perfectly fine to let relatives know that they should ask before hugging your child OR consider alternatives such as a high five or knuckle bump.

My child gets too close to others and does not seem to understand personal space boundaries. Why?

One of the unwritten rules in society involves personal space. As with any "social rule," the idea of personal space is generally learned by watching and imitating others as a baby learns to interact with those around him. However, when a child is not watching the actions of others or when he is more comfortable not looking at the person talking, he may miss important social lessons. As we get older, personal space takes on more meaning. For example, when dating, leaning into someone's personal space means something quite different than leaning into a co-worker's space during a meeting. If personal space is violated in adulthood, legal implications may result.

- Use a visual space reminder such as a hula hoop to demonstrate the appropriate amount of space your child should maintain when speaking to someone else.

- Ask children to reach out their arms. Explain that this amount of space is how much should be between them and another person.

- Review rules and make a list of possible consequences of violating personal space.

- Model the appropriate distance between two people who are communicating. Discuss different scenarios and ways to re-position the speakers to maintain an appropriate distance.

Why can't my child "read" or understand social cues, body language, sarcasm, and jokes?

Social cues and non-verbal communication can be extremely difficult for children who have autism. Since the beginning of our time, humans have used body language to show emotion and affection. You all see "emoticons" on your phone and computer. They are excellent to sum up what you're feeling without using words. Even slight facial movements show surprise, disappointment, anger, frustration, and many more. Our face has 43 muscles according to Dr. Paul Ekman.[1] Additionally, our posture, the way we move our arms/hands, and our head position all contribute to our non-verbal communication.

Sarcasm, idioms, and jokes fall within the "gray" areas of communication. Even those of us who have excellent communication skills experience difficulty interpreting sarcasm.

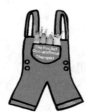

Out of the POCKET Activities

- Purchase a book of jokes and review them with your child. Discuss the ways in which the joke is or is not funny.

- Look up idioms on the internet and discuss their meanings together. I commonly draw pictures of what the idiom really means. Children who have autism learn well when there's a visual representation.

---

1   Foreman, J. (2003) "A Conversation with: Paul Ekman; The 43 Facial Muscles That Reveal Even the Most Fleeting Emotions." *The New York Times*, August 5, 2003.

- Ask your child to make a list of things he does not understand after each day OR in a journal that he carries with him.

- Make sure you inform the school of his difficulty with social skills AND reading body language. My son was sent to the principal's office once when he repeated a curse word to the teacher. He had not heard the word and did not know the true meaning. Sometimes, reviewing common curses or words which have alternate meanings can avoid an embarrassing situation.

- Play charades with each other and practice communication without verbalization.

- Use social stories about what to do when you don't understand someone. Encourage your child to ask their friends questions when they feel confused.

- Use a visual space reminder such as a hula hoop to demonstrate the appropriate amount of space your child should maintain when speaking to someone else.

- Practice communication using "scripts" such as those in a play. Use real friends' names and your child's name. Add in various situations that occur in the setting your child is in. Rehearse them often so that they can be quickly remembered when your child is in a social situation. Here's an example:

» Billy: "Hi Joey!"

» Joey: "Hello Billy, how is your day going?"

» Billy: "I have had a bad/good day."

» Joey: "What was bad/good about your day?"

» etc.

Remember that many children with communication delays get bullied due to their difficulty understanding what others truly mean. It's an important skill to learn for successful human interaction and future job success.

Chapter 9

OT in School vs. OT in an Outpatient Setting/Clinic

How are school OT and outpatient setting/clinic OT different?

When OT is prescribed in the clinic or outpatient setting, it is usually due to a suspected delay or impairment in one or many areas of activities of daily living. The delay can be a result of or in combination with a medical diagnosis. So, the delay or area of concern can be in feeding, dressing, transferring, handwriting, shoe tying, sensory processing, and so on. Most insurances require a referral from the pediatrician or specialist and then a prescription is written. This prescription is good for one calendar year. The therapist completes an evaluation to determine areas of weakness and, after review with the parent, the treatment plan is written. In the USA, the payors for therapy in outpatient settings are private insurance, state insurance, or cash payment. One-on-one sessions are usually provided. The goals of the treatment plan are frequently reviewed and the child continues to receive therapy until her progress reaches the level of expectation/goals or the child does not progress (plateaus) for a period of time. The child is then either discharged or a break from therapy is given and periodic reassessments are arranged between the caregiver, physician, and therapist.

How do I get my child's outpatient/clinic OT paid for?

If the insurance company pays for therapy, they set the rules as to the frequency and duration of therapy a child may receive. Specific insurance companies have rules and regulations as to what they will cover. In the USA, there are codes that are universally used for different diagnoses and for billing that therapists assign to each child and for the techniques the OT performs during the session. The codes are then sent with a billing form to the insurance company who then decides to pay or not to pay. Often, the OT will obtain a "prior authorization" for therapy. This means that a specific number of sessions will be approved based on the codes that are submitted for each session.

A question that I'm asked almost weekly is "Why is my insurance denying my OT?" It is critical for a caregiver—especially a caregiver of a child with special needs—to investigate the coverage of therapy *before* choosing an insurance plan. Most insurance companies STILL do not consider sensory processing/sensory integration as a "real" diagnosis and will not cover it.

Some companies feel that OT treatment techniques for sensory processing disorder are "investigational." There are many OTs and organizations that are battling with insurance companies to change this. There are even companies who do not cover OT related to the diagnosis of autism. This is changing quickly, though, as rates of autism and advocacy increase. As you investigate whether or not your insurance company will cover OT services as an outpatient, be sure to call them and request the specific codes and diagnoses to help the therapy to be covered under your specific benefits. You are your child's best advocate and knowledge is indeed power when related to coverage of OT by insurance companies.

Who pays for school OT?

The Individuals with Disability Education Act Amendment (IDEA) is the amended and retitled Public Law 94-142 in the USA. IDEA is a Federal law and gives the formal process for assessing children with disabilities and providing them with the services and programs they need for success in school. The law outlines the legal requirements for school districts to ensure that children with disabilities receive an "appropriate" education. The Americans with Disabilities Act (referred to as the ADA) is intended to prevent discrimination against children with disabilities. There is also Section 504, which is an access law that prohibits a school district from denying your child access to an educational program or educational facilities. So, the school setting is governed by Federal laws and rules.

In the school setting, Federal regulations describe physical therapy and occupational therapy as "related services," deemed necessary when they are required to assist a child with a disability to benefit from special education. IDEA rules state that the school district is responsible for providing related services and not medical services. It is only appropriate to provide PT and OT to children who qualify for special education services. These needs are agreed upon by the family and educational team and are reflected in the goals and adaptations on the child's Individual Education Plan (IEP). So, the presence of medical disabilities or injuries does not mean the child qualifies for OT services in the school system. The IEP team determines which related services a student needs. The goals and objectives in the IEP are specific to each child. The goals for school OT must advance that student's ability to succeed in the classroom. The school district or state funding such as Medicaid pays for related services.

Note: OT and PT cannot stand alone as specialized instruction under the IDEA. This means that the child must receive another special education service.

How and when does my child receive school OT?

Your child receives OT based on the frequency outlined in the IEP. The team decides together the amount and type of therapy needed. The OT does not legally have to be present at the IEP but can be if necessary. There are two types of services a school OT can provide: direct and indirect. Direct services are those times when the OT or COTA (Certified OT Assistant) has hands-on treatment with your child. This must occur in the least restrictive environment (LRE) or where students with disabilities are educated with children who are not disabled and removal from that environment is necessary based on severity of the disability. For example, your child may receive direct help from the OT on his handwriting skills when the rest of the class is involved in a handwriting exercise. The OT may work in gym class on motor coordination while the other students engage in the same gym activity. The direct services of the OT must fit into the typical schedule of the student on any given day. Indirect services include times when the OT attends meetings, collaboration, or consultation with parents, teaching staff, and other professionals working with your child at school. So, the OT is not directly working hands-on with your child during the indirect service time.

What does "educationally relevant" mean?

The OT at school uses some of the same techniques as the OT in the clinic/outpatient setting but the priorities can be different. School OT goals must be educationally relevant. Dressing, grooming, eating and drinking, organizational strategies, attention, vision, and use of adaptive equipment are all areas a school OT would work with. So, any goal set by the IEP team and carried out by the OT must directly relate to the child's school day. Scissoring, handwriting, and organizational skills are often addressed by the OT at school.

The OT completes a formal assessment and provides a written report. She should give a summary of the student's current functional level and note the student's needs relative to her participation in special education. Does the student have difficulty in the areas listed above? Does she have potential for improvement with OT intervention? How can the environment be changed to allow for the student to achieve her educational goals?

When can the school OT discharge my child?

Therapists in all settings must constantly monitor progress toward goal achievement. The OT can discharge your child when the goals have been met and the IEP team decides that no additional goals are needed to achieve the full benefit of his individual education plan. Therapy may also be discharged if therapy goals are no longer relevant to his educational goals and the child's deficits are no longer impacting his education. If someone else on the treatment team can assist the child and the expertise of the OT is no longer needed or the student has learned the strategies taught to him by the OT, he will be discharged from OT treatment. However, any time a change is made to a service for a student, the IEP must be opened and reviewed in an IEP meeting. The treatment team then assesses the changes and signs off on them. It is important to remember that in an IEP the goals are written for the child and not for the specific discipline that is working on the goal.

When can the outpatient/clinic OT discharge my child?

In the clinic, the OT completes standardized and other testing to determine goals. There does not have to be any formal meeting or IEP in place. The only team members required to participate in the clinical setting are the child, the caregiver, and the therapist. The goals are designed by the OT, but do not have to relate specifically to school areas. For example, a child's goal can be specifically for learning how to use a utensil during meal times correctly 100 percent of the time. Another goal could be that the child will demonstrate the ability to fasten buttons, zips, and snaps independently. Goals can be set for any activity of daily living (ADL) area. When goals are met and the child is functioning at age level, the child should be discharged from OT.

There are times when insurance benefits are exhausted. Some plans permit 25 visits per benefit or calendar year. When these visits are used, there are simply none left. The caregiver either has the option of paying out-of-pocket or waiting until the next benefit period. In cases such as these, the OT will assign a well-organized home therapy program. Generally most OTs are willing to provide consultation during therapy "breaks" to the family to ensure proper follow-up and completion of the program. Some US states have funding for Medicaid programs or waivers for therapy that a family is able to apply for when all other funds are exhausted. These programs require the services of a case manager. Contact your physician or local support groups in your area for additional information. You may be pleasantly surprised by the available funding if you're willing to do some digging!

Pocket Occupational Therapist Developmental Checklists

It is important that you use the developmental charts as a general guideline for development. Every child develops at his own unique pace. The experience he is given along with his pre-programming will determine how fast or slowly he meets each milestone. If you suspect that your child is not meeting milestones, share your concerns with your pediatrician. You as the caregiver know your child best. Many times throughout my career and own personal experience, someone has shared that they have discussed their child's slow progress with a doctor and was given the response, "He's just a boy, that's how it goes. He will catch up." If you feel that your doctor or therapist has not truly listened to your concerns and goals for your child, please seek a second opinion. Most times, there's nothing to worry about and your child will catch up and meet or exceed the developmental guidelines, but a caregiver's well-being is important and having the feeling of comfort is imperative to your health as well as your child's. Worry and concern are normal emotions of being a caregiver and you are your child's best advocate. It is best to learn this early on.

Developmental Checklist: Under Two Years Old

	Two Months	Six Months	One Year	Eighteen Months
Feeding	• Drinks with appropriate suck, swallow, breathe technique from bottle or breast	• Feeds self with fingers • Begins introducing solid foods • Drinks from a cup with lots of spillage	• Feeds self with fingers and is beginning fork and spoon use • Uses cup with handles, but it tips	• Spoon feeds • Uses sippy or open cup
Arm and Hand Use	• Supports himself while on his tummy with his forearms • Grasp is reflexive and not purposeful	• Grasps and brings objects to mouth • Opens hands to grasp toys • Rakes in small objects with fingers from the table	• Plays pat-a-cake • Pokes with fingers • Shakes rattles • Makes marks on paper with crayon • Uses pincer grasp (finger and thumb)	• Sits unsupported to use arms for play • Fingers move independently from each other • Removes socks
Cognitive	• Responds to faces • Pays attention to voices • Smiles responsively	• Recognizes parent's voice • Recognizes name • Smiles • Imitates "razzing" sound	• Plays peek-a-boo • Explores objects with hands and mouth • Imitates others	• May begin to refuse foods • Beginning of self-assertion • Finds comfort in familiar objects

Copyright © Cara Koscinski 2013

Developmental Checklist: Under Two Years Old cont.

	Two Months	Six Months	One Year	Eighteen Months
Visual/ Perceptual	• Shows pleasure when looking at faces • Moves eyes from side to side	• Coordinates head and eyes to move up and down	• Finds a partially hidden object • Can take object out of a container	• Points to objects you name in a book
Play Skills	• Coos and bats at toys	• Transfers a toy from hand to hand • Enjoys mirror play • Plays with feet	• Stacks rings and blocks • Turns pages of a board book • Claps hands	• Throws ball overhand • Attempts to place pieces into simple puzzles
Gross Motor	• Lifts head and neck with support of forearms while on tummy	• Rolls over • Can sit with support • Moves in and out of sitting position	• Crawls, creeps, or scoots • Walks holding on to furniture	• Walks alone • Pulls toys while walking • Climbs • Dances to music

Developmental Checklist: Two- to Five-Year-Olds

	Second Year	Third Year	Fourth Year	Fifth Year
Feeding	• Drinks without spilling • Can use a straw	• Uses fork and spoon while eating	• Pours and cuts with supervision	• Eats independently
Dressing and Bathing	• Takes off socks and shoes by end of year	• Can put on pullover, shirts, and pants • Puts on socks • Snaps • Unzips	• Buttons • Washes and dries hands	• Uses toilet on his own • Ties shoelaces • Zips • Brushes teeth
Handwriting	• Imitates a vertical and horizontal line	• Copies a circle • Copies a cross	• Draws a person with at least two body parts • Copies a square	• Draws a triangle and diagonal lines • Writes first name • Uses tripod grasp
Scissoring	• Holds scissors to snip at paper	• Cuts across paper into two pieces	• Cuts along a six-inch straight line and, by end of year, cuts a circle and square	• Cuts along a curved line and cuts out shapes

	Second Year	Third Year	Fourth Year	Fifth Year
Play Skills	• Pokes at bubbles • Builds towers of at least four blocks • Copies others' actions	• Takes turns • Completes three-piece puzzles • Plays make-believe • Rolls and pounds clay	• Plays card or board games • Can tell fantasy from reality • Catches ball	• Throws overhand ball • Knows about use of everyday objects such as money
Hand Skills	• No definite hand dominance • Turns knobs	• Screws and unscrews jar lids • Turns pages one at a time	• Colors within the lines	• Traces numbers and letters
Gross Motor	• Runs • Kicks a ball	• Walks up stairs with alternating feet	• Hops • Stands on one foot for two seconds • Rides a tricycle	• Swings • Jumps on one foot • Somersaults • Skips
Cognitive	• Sorts shapes and colors • Finds things when hidden	• Gives first name • Holds up fingers to tell age	• Sorts by shape, color, and size • Begins to understand time	• Counts to ten • Knows right from left • Is aware of gender

Developmental Checklist: Two- to Five-Year-Olds cont.

Resource Area

Catalogs and websites for products for handwriting, vision workbooks, strengthening and sensory equipment, and swings

Abilitations
www.schoolspeciality.com

Achievement Products for Children
www.achievement-products.com

Beyond Play
www.beyondplay.com

Constructive Playthings
www.cptoy.com

Differently-Abled Toy Guide from Toys-R-Us
www.toysrus.com

Educational Toys Planet
www.educationaltoysplanet.com

Flag House
www.flaghouse.com

Fun and Function
www.funandfuction.com

Kid Companions (wearable/chewable jewelry for oral-input)
www.kidcompanions.com

Pacific Pediatric Supply
www.pacificpediatricsupply.com

Pocket Full of Therapy
www.pfot.com

Pro-Ed
www.proediric.com

Route2Greatness
www.route2greatness.com

Sensory Edge
www.sensoryedge.com

Sensory Interventions
www.sensoryinterventions.com

SensoryStreet
www.sensorystreet.com

Sensory University Toy Company
www.sensoryuniversity.com

Southpaw
www.southpawenterprises.com

TFH Special Needs Toys
www.specialneedstoys.com

Therapy Shoppe
www.therapyshoppe.com

Sites and catalogs for clothing and weighted blankets

DreamCatcher Weighted Blankets
www.weightedblanket.net

EZ Socks
www.kidssocks.com

Fun and Function
www.funandfunction.com

Quilted Illusions
www.quiltedillusions.com

SPIO Pressure Garments
www.spioworks.com

Soft Clothing
www.softclothing.net

The Sensory Gallery
www.thesensorygallery.com

Sew Sensory (Custom Weighted Vests)
www.sewsensory.com

Websites with printables and other activities

Do2Learn
www.dotolearn.com

edHelper.com
www.edhelper.com

funbrain
www.funbrain.com

The Kidz Club
www.thekidzclub.com

KidPrintables.com
www.kidprintables.com

Starfall.com
www.starfall.com

Educational advocacy, information, and rights for children with disabilities

Global Autism Collaboration
www.autism.org

National Center for Learning Disabilities
www.ncld.org

Nolo's IEP Guide: Learning Disabilities by Attorney
Lawrence M. Siegel
www.nolo.com

OASIS
www.aspergersyndrome.org

The Council of Parent Attorneys and Advocates
www.copaa.org

Wrightslaw
www.wrightslaw.com

Note: For more information or additional resources
visit Cara Koscinski's website: *www.pocketot.com*

International occupational therapy organizations

USA

AOTA

American Occupational Therapy Association

www.aota.org

UK

BAOT/COT

British Association of Occupational Therapists and College of Occupational Therapists

www.cot.co.uk

Australia and New Zealand

Occupational Therapy Council (Australia and New Zealand) Inc.

www.cotrb.com.au

Canada

CAOT

Canadian Association of Occupational Therapists

www.caot.ca

South Africa

OTASA

Occupational Therapy Association of South Africa

www.otasa.org.za

World

WFOT

World Federation of Occupational Therapists

www.wfot.org

Index